you don't
need plastic
surgery

also by the authors

Everett M. Lautin, M.D., FACR, Suzanne M. Levine, DPM, and Kathryn Lance:
The Botox Book: What You Need to Know About America's Most Popular Cosmetic Treatment

Everett M. Lautin, M.D.:
Genitourinary Radiology: A Multimodality Approach

Suzanne M. Levine:
Your Feet Don't Have to Hurt
My Feet Are Killing Me
50 Ways to Ease Foot Pain
Walk if Off

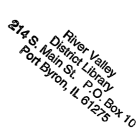

you don't need plastic surgery

the doctors' guide to youthful looks with no surgery, no pain, no downtime

Everett M. Lautin, M.D., FACR, Suzanne M. Levine, D.P.M.
and Kathryn Lance

M. Evans and Company, Inc.
New York

DISCLAIMER

This publication is designed to provide accurate and authoritative information in regard to the subject matter covered. It is sold with the understanding that the publisher is not engaged in rendering professional services. If legal, accounting, medical, psychological, or any other expert assistance is required, the services of a competent professional person should be sought.

The information, ideas, procedures, and suggestions contained in this book are not intended to replace the services of a trained healthcare professional or to serve as a replacement for professional medical advice and care or as a substitute for any treatment prescribed by your physician. Matters regarding an individual's health often require medical supervision. A physician or health-care professional should be consulted regarding the use of any of the ideas, procedures, suggestions, or drug therapies in this book. Any application of the information set forth in this book is at the reader's discretion. The author and publisher hereby specifically disclaim any and all liability arising directly or indirectly from the use or application of any of the products, ideas, procedures, drug therapies, or suggestions contained in this book and any errors, omissions, and inaccuracies in the information contained herein.

Trade names are included for identification purposes only, and are not intended to endorse the product.

M. Evans and Company, Inc.
216 East 49th Street
New York, New York 10017

Library of Congress Cataloguing-in-Publication Data

Lautin, Everett M.
    You Don't Need Plastic Surgery / Everett Lautin, Suzzane M. Levine, and Kathryn Lance
        p. cm.
    Includes index
    ISBN 1-59077-000-5
        1. Beauty, Personal. 2. Face—Care and hygiene. 3. Skin—Care and hygiene. I. Levine, Suzanne M. II. Lance, Kathryn. III. Title
    RL87.L35 2003
    646.7'2—dc21

                                                                2002192808

Printed in the United States of America

9 8 7 6 5 4 3 2 1

dedications

Everett M. Lautin: I dedicate this book to my colleague and friend, Suzanne M. Levine, D.P.M., for her inspiration; to my father, Arthur Lautkin, M.D., for teaching me the power of logical thinking; to my mother, Fredda B. Lautkin, for her support and teaching me the value of a proper work ethic; and to my children, Douglas and Dana, for being there.

Suzanne M. Levine: I dedicate this book to my colleague and friend, Everett M. Lautin, M.D., for his intelligence and originality, and to my children, Marisa and Heather, for their support.

contents

acknowledgments

We are grateful to all the beauty and fashion editors whose critical aesthetic skills and insights have proved invaluable in guiding and fine-tuning our aesthetic senses. In particular, we acknowledge: Anna Wintour, Amy Astley, Jillian Demling, and André Talley of *Vogue* magazine; DiDi Gluck of *Marie Claire*; Sallie Brady of *Concorde Magazine*; and Gena Way of *US Weekly*. We also thank Katie Couric, Emiko Tate, and Betsy Alexander of *Today*; Florence Henderson of *Later Today* and her beautiful daughter Barbara Chase; and Karen Harris of *NBC News*; Susan Ducher of *NBC Weekend Today*; Matt Strauss at *The View*; High Voltage, who helped transform us, and Donna Lapkin, whose aesthetic sensibilities and courage guided us.

We acknowledge the untiring efforts of Kathryn Lance in providing background research and compiling this book in a thorough yet expeditious manner.

We acknowledge the consummate editing skills of PJ Dempsey and George de Kay of M. Evans Publishing, and our agent Linda Konner for making this book possible.

We acknowledge the assistance of the many people who contributed information to this book, including: Joseph Georghy, M.D., Andrew Wong, M.D., Ana Vila Joya, M.D., Ellen Fischl Bodner and James Shaoul, M.D., Vivienne Mackinder, Alan Matarasso, M.D., Karen E. Burke, M.D., Zoe Diana Draelos, M.D., Deborah Hardwick, Eva To, Marc Lowenberg, D.D.S., Denise Chaplin, Daniel Hamermesh, Ph.D., James J. Romano, M.D., and Howard M. Shapiro, M.D.

We acknowledge our dedicated staff: Wincess Elias, Jinet Delgado, Louise Russo, Toni Lopez Morales, and Chloe.

And, of course, we acknowledge all of our wonderful patients, who provided a beautiful canvas on which we could work.

you don't
need plastic
surgery

introduction

the good news about good looks

D id you ever wonder why so many models, actors, and TV personalities look so great in their middle and later years? Maybe you assumed that these men and women had undergone plastic surgery—even those who denied it. These days, the chances are good that these great-looking people haven't had any surgery at all; rather, they have taken advantage of the latest technological advances in rejuvenating treatments.

These products and procedures are not secret, but most people assume they are out of reach for all but the rich and famous. The good news is that all these treatments are affordable and they are becoming more so every day. For the cost of a health club membership, for example, you can have several nonsurgical procedures that will restore a firm and unblemished appearance to the skin on your face which will last for years. The price of a business suit can get you a treatment that will relax and smooth out the lines in your forehead and around your eyes. A six-month supply of a prescription skin cream that fades blemishes and fine wrinkles costs less than a facial at most spas. The bottom line is that today there is no reason to look old unless you want to.

It sounds unbelievable, but these new techniques and products can virtually eliminate crow's feet; deeper furrows between the brows and around the mouth; blotches and uneven skin tone; rosacea; sagging jowls and "turkey neck;" thickened, discolored nails; and even worn and discolored teeth. All of these once inevitable signs of aging can now be delayed, reduced, or even eliminated quickly and *without any surgery and with minimal or no recovery time.*

A generation or two ago, fifty was the start of old age. When your grandparents were through raising a family, they were pretty much through with life. They began to dress in drab, shapeless "old people's" clothes. Their hair turned gray and stayed that way. Their skin wrinkled, their toenails turned yellow and thick, and they headed for the rocking chair.

What a difference a few years make!

Today, fifty is the start of middle age, a time that is expected to be vigorous and productive. Many of us are starting new careers or embarking on travel adventures. Others are parents—for the second or even the first time. We dress to look shapely, chic, and sharp—drab and shapeless is now inappropriate. Our hair is any color we want it to be. We are much more likely to be touring the country on a mountain bike than smiling sardonically in a rocking chair.

For many of us, looking old simply isn't an option. Our jobs often require us to project a youthful, vigorous image. While it may be true that "beauty is only skin deep," the skin is the first part of you that everyone sees—and judges you by.

As recently as fifteen years ago, the only way to get rid of wrinkles was to have a facelift and the only way to get rid of splotches was to have a deep peel. Both of these procedures are very expensive and carry numerous potential side effects, such as scarring, and even in the best cases can result in a taut, asymmetrical, and unnatural appearance. Today, there are dozens of things you can do to maintain or regain youthful, smooth, unwrinkled skin.

Without ever visiting a doctor, you can start—right now!—to improve your appearance and look younger, healthier, and more relaxed. There are products and regimens out there, some inexpensive, that can ameliorate the ravages of time and help restore a youthful appearance. You don't need a facelift to have smooth, relatively wrinkle-free skin, even into old age. You don't need false teeth to have a bright and winning smile. And you don't need liposuction to achieve or regain a slim, trim, youthful figure.

If you do decide that you want a medical solution to your aging appearance, there are many modern treatments that are far more effective, less risky, and less costly than the old-fashioned facelifts and extreme peels. Furthermore, many of these treatments offer instant results that get even better over time. Our years of experience with these treatments in our *Institute Beauté* has convinced us and our clients that an ageless, time-defying look is no longer the provenance of the wealthy, or of those rare souls with age-defying genes.

Our many clients, both celebrities and the rest of us, have proved to themselves that the years after youth can be not only the most productive, but the most attractive as well. We will introduce you to these clients and let you hear their stories so you can see for yourself that growing older needn't mean growing less attractive.

Take Audrey, a fifty-something real-estate saleswoman, who admits that as a young woman she worshipped the sun, with winters in Miami Beach, island-hopping in the Hawaiian Islands and the Caribbean, and summers in the Hamptons. When she came to us, she was an attractive auburn-haired dynamo with dry, wrinkled, spotted skin that made her look years older than her calendar age. After only four CoolTouch laser treatments over a period of three months, coupled with several injectable implants in her deepest wrinkles, Audrey's skin is again youthful and smooth. "The results are amazing," she says. "I don't look like I did when I was thirty, or even thirty-five, but I'll bet that at least ten years have been erased from my skin. And in only three months!"

Another of our clients is High Voltage, the personal trainer and nutrition expert whom you may have seen on *The Today Show* and CNN, and whose abilities as a fitness guru were praised by Katie Couric when she was a guest on *The Tonight Show.* When she came to us, High Voltage was resigned to receiving her *third* expensive and painful facelift, as the previous ones had inevitably loosened. "I was lucky," she declared. "My facelifts hadn't really harmed me up to that point. But I learned from Dr. Lautin and Dr. Levine that the older you get, the worse it looks when you pull back the skin."

What the fifty-five-year-old Voltage needed—along with most of our clients in their mid-fifties to sixties—was not to have the skin stretched back, but rather to have the face plumped out, to restore the natural padding of youth. We recommended a few treatments with CoolTouch Laser. "It sounded ridiculous," Voltage admitted. "But the doctors explained to me how CoolTouch stimulates the body to produce its own collagen, which would last for years.

My face filled out and started looking great again. It was like gaining weight in my face without having to gain in my butt."

Voltage also received a few treatments of injectable implants in the deepest wrinkles around her mouth area. "I'd had injections of bovine collagen in the past," she said. "But they always got lumpy and only lasted a few weeks. These are soft and natural, like my own skin."

As for the final results, "I looked so much better immediately," she said. "And it just keeps getting better."

By the way, cosmetic improvement is no longer just for women. Many of our most satisfied clients are men.

Tom Fuchs, a fifty-one-year-old real estate owner and entrepreneur, had minimal work done (CoolTouch and injectable implants) to erase the wrinkles around his eyes and on his brow, and to smooth his aging skin. "The results are subtle," he admits three months later. "Women's heads aren't yet turning in the street. But I've been told that the effects increase over time. And I definitely seem to look better and more youthful."

For a more dramatic male success story, see the box on page 6.

• • •

We realize that not everyone wants to receive medical treatment, even the minimally invasive procedures we offer at *Institute Beauté*. The good news is that for those who wish to age naturally, but with a healthier, more youthful look, there are a number of preparations available—some over-the-counter, others by prescription—that not only help retard the signs of aging, but that can also smooth and clarify already-damaged skin.

In the next pages, we will tell you everything you need to know about the things you can do now to retard the signs of aging, literally from head to toe, and feel better and be healthier in the bargain. We'll sort out the confusing terminology and explain exactly what Botox, YAG-erbium, chemical peels, and other cutting-edge treatments do. We'll tell you about the skin preparations you can use, their names, and how to use them. We'll also tell you how to beautify aging teeth and nails, how to have sexy hands and feet, and how to age-proof your body. Our intention is to offer you a complete and detailed overview of what's available to improve and maintain your good looks literally from head to toe.

In this book you will learn about:

- Over-the-counter and prescription skin products that actually do what they promise
- New cosmetics that can disguise and enhance your own natural looks
- Why it's never too late to smooth over acne scars
- How to reduce active acne and reduce new acne scars
- State-of-the-art laser treatments that tighten your skin, including the "lunchtime" lift that takes only minutes but erases years
- Light chemical peels and microdermabrasion that resurface your skin
- How to get rid of unwanted hair painlessly, permanently, and quickly
- Botox, the poison for wrinkles and excess sweating
- Simple exercises you can do to improve the tone of your face and body
- How to beautify your battered feet
- How to erase spider veins on your legs and broken capillaries on your face
- How to have an "attitude lift" that will enable you to look and feel years younger

We'll tell you everything you need to know, from how to choose and use the best rejuvenating products to how to choose a doctor; the multiple treatment options for every situation and the advantages and drawbacks to each. We want you to think of this book as your complete consumer guide to maintaining a youthful appearance and vibrant health well into your later years. We want to be your advocates against time.

> **Authors' note:** Although all the treatments we describe in this book can improve the appearance of both men and women, most of our examples feature women because at present many more women than men take advantage of these rejuvenating procedures and products.

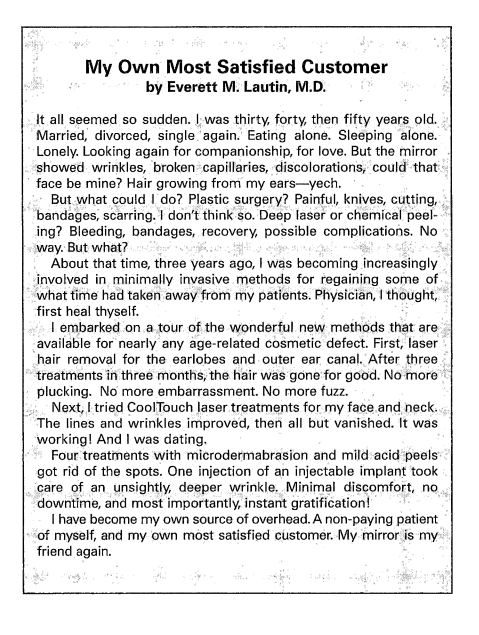

My Own Most Satisfied Customer
by Everett M. Lautin, M.D.

It all seemed so sudden. I was thirty, forty, then fifty years old. Married, divorced, single again. Eating alone. Sleeping alone. Lonely. Looking again for companionship, for love. But the mirror showed wrinkles, broken capillaries, discolorations, could that face be mine? Hair growing from my ears—yech.

But what could I do? Plastic surgery? Painful, knives, cutting, bandages, scarring. I don't think so. Deep laser or chemical peeling? Bleeding, bandages, recovery, possible complications. No way. But what?

About that time, three years ago, I was becoming increasingly involved in minimally invasive methods for regaining some of what time had taken away from my patients. Physician, I thought, first heal thyself.

I embarked on a tour of the wonderful new methods that are available for nearly any age-related cosmetic defect. First, laser hair removal for the earlobes and outer ear canal. After three treatments in three months, the hair was gone for good. No more plucking. No more embarrassment. No more fuzz.

Next, I tried CoolTouch laser treatments for my face and neck. The lines and wrinkles improved, then all but vanished. It was working! And I was dating.

Four treatments with microdermabrasion and mild acid peels got rid of the spots. One injection of an injectable implant took care of an unsightly, deeper wrinkle. Minimal discomfort, no downtime, and most importantly, instant gratification!

I have become my own source of overhead. A non-paying patient of myself, and my own most satisfied customer. My mirror is my friend again.

PART ONE

making the
most of your
skin

–

chapter one
looking great at any age

There's an old saying that youth is wasted on the young. The implication is that the combination of health, good looks, and energy youth confers isn't really appreciated until later in life when that health, beauty, and energy are on the wane. While there's admittedly a bit of truth in this saying, we'd like to amend it: youth is possible at any age.

It's true that you'll never again have the innocence and fresh beauty you possessed at twenty, but it's also true that you'll never again have the problems you had then. What you *can* have now is the energy and vibrant health—with the ageless looks to go with them—that are optimum at any age.

In the bad old days of even ten years ago, middle-aged men and women who wanted to change their looks had to submit to severe procedures—facelifts or harsh chemical peels—that often left their faces asymmetrical and unnatural-looking. These procedures required a long recovery period of weeks to months, actually disrupted the blood supply to the face, and sometimes caused nerve damage. Furthermore, because they generally didn't address the causes of aging looks, these measures only temporarily disguised the problem.

While it's true that gravity works its inevitable mischief on all parts of our bodies, it's not the primary cause of facial sag; rather, loss of the skin's elasticity and support (provided by elastin and collagen), combined with a loss of padding in the form of fat, leads to deeper wrinkles and a gaunt, slack facial appearance.

the down side of a facelift

Instead of restoring padding or encouraging the growth of new collagen, surgical facelifts and deep peels basically do one of two things: burn off the top layers of the skin (harsh chemical peel), or pull the skin tight (facelift). Burning off the top layers of the skin certainly helps eliminate superficial blemishes—age spots and fine wrinkles—but it does little for the muscle-wrinkles (also known as dynamic wrinkles) caused by repeated facial movement. Moreover, though this method eliminates superficial imperfections, the skin is severely damaged in the process, a fact often obvious to the patient and everyone who sees him for a long time.

Pulling the skin tight through a conventional facelift flattens out the deeper, dynamic wrinkles and tightens sags, but at the cost of a stretched-out, unnatural, wide-eyed appearance. Instead of being filled in, deeper wrinkles, including the unattractive furrows from nose to chin, often accompanied by jowls, are simply pulled tight, like smoothing a bed sheet, which actually distorts the face.

Even worse for those who undergo these extreme procedures, the aging process still continues, resulting in a worse appearance as they grow older. In our opinion, people in their seventies and eighties who have never undergone plastic surgery age far better than those who had those invasive procedures done when they were younger. The adhesions from the scar tissue along the hairline where the cuts were made don't move, but as the rest of the face continues gradually to sag, the result is an unattractive and unnatural-looking asymmetry.

the goal of looking good at any age

The problem with surgical procedures is that they try to achieve a young look as opposed to a youthful look, which is our aim. Men and women in their fifties simply cannot look like thirty-year-olds. Instead of the look of youth, the new procedures strive for an *ageless* look, one that creates the optimum appearance possible no matter what a person's calendar age.

This is done through a combination of the latest scientific products and techniques. Combined with a regimen of home care, the treatments are long-lasting and totally natural-looking. No, we can't restore your youth—but we can help you be a more beautiful you.

THE FOUR "MAGIC" PROCEDURES

It's not magic, but good hard science that has finally come to understand the primary causes of aging looks and found methods to address them. Now we'd like to give you an idea of what's possible with four basic "magic" procedures, used alone or in combination with each other and some other treatments.

1. **Microdermabrasion.** This popular procedure offers the results of a peel without the downtime. Microdermabrasion employs a controlled fine mist of microscopic aluminum oxide (or sodium chloride) crystals that are sprayed on the top layers of skin, causing exfoliation (removal of the outer layers of dead skin). This is immediately vacuumed away, thereby gradually diminishing fine lines, wrinkles, acne scars, and discoloration. Microdermabrasion requires no anesthesia and only takes about thirty minutes, one reason it's often referred to as the "lunchtime" peel.

   For optimum results, five to ten treatments at about one-week intervals are recommended and can be combined with a mild acid peel. Some people are so pleased with the results that they have regular treatments every few weeks for extended periods of time. After the initial series is completed, touch-up treatments are indicated as a beauty maintenance practice. Some people even find it relaxing.

2. **Botox.** Botox is a product made from a toxin (made by botulinum bacteria) that relaxes muscles. When purified and made safe for cosmetic use, Botox weakens the muscles that pull on the skin to create dynamic wrinkles, such as frown lines, and brow furrows. This causes the wrinkles to disappear naturally

after a few days. Each Botox treatment lasts four to six months, and over time may need to be repeated less often. This "magical" product can also be used to relax the platysma muscles in the neck, helping to ease "turkey neck," the ugly aging lines and folds that often occur there. To learn how Botox can enhance your appearance, see chapter 4.

3. **Injectable implants.** Miraculous space-age products, such as Artecoll, Reviderm, Restylane, Rofilan, Perlane, New Fill, and others can be used to fill in deep lines and wrinkles, as well as acne scars. Unlike the old-fashioned collagen or fat injections, these new injectables are longer-lasting or permanent, and carry little risk of allergic reaction or rejection. For more information on these beauty-enhancing products, see chapter 5.

4. **CoolTouch Laser.** This is one of the most magical of all the tricks in the modern doctor's "magic bag." One of a number of laser tools designed to enhance the beauty of the skin, the CoolTouch Laser uses a YAG-erbium laser beam (using a crystal made from yttrium, aluminum, garnet, and erbium) to target the deeper layers of your skin (about 0.5 millimeters deep), while a cooling spray protects the skin surface and allows the laser to pass harmlessly through the outer layers. (This is a non-ablative laser, meaning it does not affect nor remove the outer layer of skin.)

    CoolTouch actually rejuvenates your skin from the inside out, stimulating the formation of collagen, the structural material that gives skin its plumpness and resilience. Depending upon the areas treated and how many passes are performed with the laser, each treatment of the face lasts 15 to 30 minutes; three to five treatments at a minimum of 3-week intervals are recommended initially. While most people experience some very transient burning, especially on the upper lip, this is over in seconds. Not only is there no recovery time, most people find that the minimal swelling that lasts one or two days after the treatment smoothes out the wrinkles and looks great, a preview of the final results. New collagen continues to be produced for months after your treatment, with gradual ongoing improvement.

    The results may be subtle at first, but they become dramatic as time passes, reaching a maximum result at about six months after the final treatment that should last for years. Superficial wrinkles disappear. As the skin begins to fill out from the inside, that aging, gaunt look disappears. CoolTouch can be used on any part of your body—even the bottoms of your feet (see chapter 17)—to restore some of the natural padding that has disappeared with age.

We find that one or more of these treatments, often in combination with a variety of topical preparations, both prescription and over the counter, can significantly reduce the following signs of aging.

how we can help

Discolored skin with fine wrinkles. These are among the most common signs of aging skin, and, depending on how much time you have spent in the sun, can begin as early as your thirties. Those dreaded brown spots, slangily referred to as "age spots" or "liver spots" (technically, seborrheic keratoses), occur when the skin, trying to protect itself from ongoing damage from ultraviolet light, releases melanin (the dark pigment that protects the skin) unevenly. The fine lines are the result of the skin's loss of elasticity and a diminished ability to hold moisture.

Sarah, a Scarsdale homemaker in her mid-forties, was nervous when we first met with her. An extremely attractive natural blonde, Sarah was impeccably groomed and coiffed, but her skin showed the telltale signs of aging: fine wrinkles on her cheeks and at the corners of her eyes, as well as brown spots on her cheeks and above her lips.

"My husband tells me I look good," she told us. "But when I look in the mirror, all I see are the wrinkles and spots."

We prepared a complete treatment plan for Sarah, beginning with a very mild beta peel (salicylic acid) to remove the top damaged layers of skin, followed by microdermabrasion.

"I couldn't believe it," Sarah said. "After the very first treatment, my face looked smoother and healthier."

We recommended a series of ten treatments over a period of several weeks, in conjunction with CoolTouch laser (three to five treatments about three to five weeks apart) to help smooth out the wrinkles by stimulating Sarah's skin to make new collagen. After only seven weeks, Sarah was ecstatic. "The spots are almost gone," she told us. "My husband gets jealous again when other men look at me at the Galleria Mall."

Deep furrows between the eyes and around the mouth. The furrows that many of us develop between the eyes and on the forehead are prime examples of dynamic wrinkles, caused by overuse of the "frown" muscles. The deep lines around the mouth are more complex. They are caused by a combination of muscle movement and the loss of fat padding under the surface of the skin, and are often associated with smoking. When that lost padding is replaced with injectable implants in tandem with the CoolTouch laser, a long-lasting natural and youthful appearance is restored.

Carole, age fifty-two, teaches art to schoolchildren. Concerned about the lines on her forehead and around her mouth, she came to us for help. "I'm happy with myself the way I am," she told us. "But I'm an artist. I'm very visual. I dress nicely and I want a face to match."

We began with Botox injections to reduce the furrows on Carole's forehead, then followed with CoolTouch to the whole facial area and injectable implants to smooth out the lines around the mouth and the deeper furrows that extended from the corners of the nose to the corners of the mouth (the nasolabial folds).

After the first treatment, Carole was amazed. The fine lines were totally gone and the skin on her face plumped up. As time passed, the results pleased Carole even more. "Before the treatments I looked *good* for my age. Now I look *better*. The teachers at school are always telling me how good I look. And the kids noticed too. I still can't believe there was no cutting and no pain."

Turkey neck. As we age, the platysma muscles in the skin of our neck weaken and separate into strands, which create those ugly vertical cords in men and women. Thinning of the skin and loss of fat, collagen, and elastin around the neck add to the unattractive appearance.

Although it is still a relatively new procedure, Botox injections can greatly improve the appearance of the neck by relaxing the platysma muscles and keeping them from separating into strings. CoolTouch laser, to plump up the skin on the neck, in concert with injectable implants, also helps to correct this unfortunate sign of aging.

Maria, a health professional, is a natural beauty who has had regular microdermabrasion treatments to keep her already-beautiful complexion flawless. As she aged, Maria added occasional laser treatments to stimulate her own collagen and prevent her minimal wrinkles from worsening. When she reached her mid-fifties, she began to develop a stringy, cordy look in her long, graceful neck. With Botox injections to the platysma muscles followed by CoolTouch applications to the skin of her neck, her neck was restored to its smooth and elegant appearance.

Tired, gaunt look. In addition to wrinkles and age spots, the effects of aging can often be more general, leading to a look of tiredness and gauntness. Although all the treatments we recommend are prescribed for specific problems, their effects are far-reaching and result in an overall improvement in appearance.

Anna, a busy executive in her mid-fifties, had two CoolTouch laser treatments followed by microdermabrasion, literally on her lunch hour. Though she received numerous compliments from clients and friends on how relaxed and healthy she looked, she wasn't sure of the results until she visited us several months later and saw her "before" picture.

Catherine came in because she was tired of being single and wanted to start dating again. "I thought about a facelift," she told us, "but I have friends who've had them and I hate that glossy, stretched-out look. Plus I don't want to be cut."

Because her aging signs were still minimal, we recommended the CoolTouch laser for her face, neck, and hands, coupled with injectable implants to the deep lines along the outside of her mouth (in medspeak, her nasolabial folds). Catherine was pleased with the results immediately. As her body continued to produce new collagen in the treated areas, her appearance also continued to improve. "My skin keeps looking younger," she said. "My friends are all asking me why I look so good. 'Who is your surgeon?' they say. 'No surgery,'" I hold them. I still haven't met that new 'he,' but men are again looking at me and I have some prospects."

Thin lips and smoker's wrinkles As subcutaneous padding disappears with age, our lips become thinner and less sensual-looking. For those who started out with relatively thin lips, the mouth can almost seem to disappear.

In the past, lips were often injected with collagen, which plumped them out, but its effects were short-lived and it sometimes caused allergic reactions. Today, we combine the CoolTouch laser with injections of newer, nonallergic materials for a long-lasting and natural-looking increase in plumpness. This combination also smoothes out those unattractive wrinkles and lines in the area above the upper lip. Microdermabrasion can be of benefit here as well. Botox is also sometimes used to relax the overactive muscles and prevent the lines from returning.

Carla, a senior research analyst at a major New York brokerage house, thrives on the fast track. Now 42, and with a trim figure that still turns heads, Carla became concerned with the wrinkles that seemed to suddenly appear around her eyes and mouth.

"I quit smoking five years ago," she told us, "But I guess smoking combined with all the stress to cause the wrinkles. I hate the way the lipstick bleeds into the lines above my upper lip. And now my upper lip is getting thinner. I think it makes me look harsh."

For the smoker's wrinkles, we recommended four treatments with the CoolTouch laser, four weeks apart, and injectable implants around the lips, which enhanced her thin upper lip and helped reduce the wrinkles.

Carla looked better immediately, and after three months she was thrilled. "I again like what I see when I look in the mirror," she says. "It's a successful businesswoman who looks like she's in her early to mid thirties."

● ๑ ๑

In addition to the specific problems we've mentioned here, the modern doctor's bag of "magic" techniques can also address other skin problems associated with aging, as well as those that can occur at any age, such as double chin, that jowly look, unwanted hair, and old acne scars. In the next chapters, we'll give you an overview of your skin and how various treatments affect it, as well as details on each of the procedures and products (some over-the-counter) that we recommend.

chapter two

what's your skin type?

D id you ever notice that some people, usually those with darker skin, seem to age much more slowly than their paler counterparts? As if to make up for this unfair advantage, however, darker-skinned people often have more problems with skin blemishes, such as acne and visible scarring, including keloid scars (an enlarged scar that projects above the skin surface).

Dermatologists classify skin into six different types (see the Fitzpatrick Scale that follows), depending on the amount of melanin, the dark pigment that gives skin and hair their color, and whether the skin tans or burns in the sun. The more melanin you have, the more protected you are from the sun, but the more likely you are to have certain skin problems and also more difficulty achieving results from some rejuvenating treatments. See our cautions for dark skin in the discussions of specific treatments, especially those for lasers and peels.

It's helpful to know your own type as a guide to some of the best procedures and products for your personal skin rejuvenation regimen.

the fitzpatrick scale of skin types		
type	**description**	**tanning capabilities**
I	Light-skinned	Never tans, always sunburns.
II	Light-skinned	Can achieve a light tan with careful sunning, but easily sunburns.
III	Light- to medium-skinned	Tans well, but can still get sunburned.
IV	Medium-skinned	Tans well and rarely sunburns.
V	Brown-skinned.	Tans well, sledom sunburns, but can burn after prolonged exposure to the sun. Includes Asians, Orientals, Native Americans, olive skin.
VI	Black-skinned	Deeply pigmented, burns after prolonged exposure to sun. Predominately African ancestry, certain Indians.

inside the skin

You probably know that your skin is composed of three layers: the epidermis, dermis, and subcutaneous layers. Each of these layers is in turn composed of many more layers of cells. The outer layer, the one you see, is the epidermis, which is made up of tightly packed dead skin cells. These cells are constantly sloughing off and just as constantly being replaced from the layers of cells beneath them. The main function of the epidermis is to provide protection from the outside world.

The middle, thickest layer of skin, the dermis, is where specialized cells called fibroblasts produce collagen and elastin, the connective tissues that provide support and structure to the skin, as well as give it the elasticity of youth. The dermis, with its thick scaffolding of collagen, also helps protect the body from mechanical injury and, as a bonus, stores moisture.

The bottom layer of skin, the subcutaneous layer, contains fat for padding

How Spanish Women Keep Themselves Beautiful
by Ana Vila Joya, M.D., Madrid, Spain

First and foremost, all Spanish women take care of their beauty on the inside. They pay attention to healthy nutrition, eating balanced and natural foods, including whole grains, fresh fruits and vegetables, fish, chicken, and some meat. They also take supplements of vitamins and minerals. We call this the Mediterranean diet.

Spanish women also care about their looks on the outside, but many of them are afraid of surgery. They worry about complications and don't want to take a chance on scarring. They also don't want to wait weeks for a treatment to heal. For this reason, more and more of them come to clinics like ours that offer excellent and immediate results without side effects.

My experience is that these women are up on the latest treatments. It is common for our patients to ask for injectable fillers to smooth out wrinkles and lines. We also offer Botox and Dysport [a European form of Botox] as well, to give the effect of a facelift without surgery.

I firmly believe that with attention to health and a little bit of health, every woman can improve her appearance and image.

and supports the nerves and blood vessels that nourish the skin. Oil and sweat glands, as well as hair follicles, originate in this layer.

natural skin renewal

When you're young, your skin constantly renews itself. Fibroblasts continually produce new collagen and elastin and the upper layers are constantly replenished, providing a fairly thick, resilient outer skin. With age, alas, all phases of this self-renewal slow down. At age fifty, your skin is actually replaced only one third as quickly as it is at age twenty.

Not only do production of collagen and the inner fat padding diminish, and the constant replenishment of the outer layers slow, damaged proteins begin to accumulate within the skin cells. Oil production also diminishes, leading to dryness. The result is skin that is thinner, less vibrant, and more easily damaged. It is also, usually, wrinkled, discolored, and old-looking.

What to do? For years, the bottom line has been to cover it up or take more drastic measures, such as deep peels. Although the outer dead layer can be made to look better by increasing moisture and removing superficial blemishes, actual skin renewal can only occur in the deeper, living layers of the skin, the dermis and the subcutaneous level.

RENEWAL PROCEDURES

Most common skin renewal procedures, such as dermabrasion, lasers, and deep-working peels are actually a form of controlled damage. The way they work is to injure the deeper layers of skin. The body responds as it does to any injury, by creating new tissues, including collagen and new skin cells.

Techniques such as CoolTouch laser treatments minimize damage to the skin. The light from the CoolTouch Laser, for example, penetrates about half a millimeter, where it stimulates the fibroblasts in the dermis of the skin, inducing them to create new collagen and elastin. Microdermabrasion accelerates the sloughing off of the dead outer layers of skin cells, revealing the natural, fresher layers underneath. Botox works by weakening the muscles that pull on the skin and create wrinkles, while injectable implants replace the diminished fat and collagen layers underlying the skin (they also stimulate collagen formation), filling in wrinkles and restoring youthful plumpness.

RENEWAL CREAMS AND LOTIONS

Most cosmetics, creams, and lotions, though they may make your skin temporarily look better by adding moisture or through optical illusions (for example, changing the way the light is reflected off of and absorbed by the surface of the skin), can't make any overall difference in your skin's health or appearance because they remain on the skin's surface and do not penetrate the deeper layers.

Special Cautions for Dark Skin

If you have naturally darker skin (type IV or higher, see The Fitzpatrick Scale on p. 18), your complexion will look good far longer than the skin of your light-skinned friends. In fact, the darker your skin, the more youthful it will appear as you age. On the downside, however, many of the products and procedures detailed in this book may not work as well for you; worse, they may cause unsightly changes in your pigmentation.

A particular problem for those with skin of type IV and higher is laser treatments, which can easily result not only in uneven pigmentation, but can even cause burns. Exceptions to this difficulty are the Lyra laser, for hair removal and the treatment of spider veins (for more information, see chapters 6 and 15), and CoolTouch II laser treatments, which can also be used for a variety of conditions without affecting pigmentation.

Products that are also likely to cause problems are alpha-hydroxy and glycolic acids; these can stimulate your melanocytes, the pigment-producing cells, to produce more melanin, leading to dark spots on your skin. This reaction does not occur with everyone, but it is a possibility to be aware of. Also problematic for some people with darker or olive skin color is tretinoin (Renova).

The best wrinkle-reducers for dark skin are retinol (over-the-counter) creams and Kinerase, which reportedly has no effect on pigmented skin. Mandelic acid, a less irritating form of alpha-hydroxy acid, is said to work well on dark skin. Copper-containing preparations such as Neova are also good for dark skin, and can help promote the growth of new collagen if used daily.

For more information on each of these treatments and products, see chapters 3 and 10, as well as Appendix B for web addresses.

Products that claim to contain collagen, for example, can't possibly augment your own collagen, which is found in the middle layer of skin. Collagen molecules are simply too large to pass passively through the protective layer of dead cells that make up the outer skin. Even if these molecules could somehow reach the middle layer, there is no way they could hook up with your natural collagen, and thus no way they could increase your skin's firmness or elasticity. That can only be done by the collagen and elastin that are produced naturally, induced to proliferate by CoolTouch laser or similar treatments (see chapter 6), or directly injected beneath the outer layers of the skin.

Just as creams and lotions can't penetrate the outer layers of skin, moisturizers don't really moisturize. Rather, they improve the waterproofing ability of the top layer of skin and help to prevent moisture loss. Some compounds, known as humectants, actually attract outside moisture to your skin, but again this moisture is only "skin deep"—confined to the epidermal layers of dead cells—and doesn't affect the deeper, living layers.

This doesn't mean that all cosmetic preparations are worthless. On the contrary, moisturizers can certainly keep your skin looking and feeling better. Furthermore, some medical-strength preparations, such as the active ingredients in Renova and Kinerase, and some antioxidants, most notably Vitamin C, actually penetrate to the deeper layers of the skin and stimulate cell renewal (see chapter 3). Other topical preparations that contain antioxidants (such as vitamins C and E and green tea extract) can help protect the skin from some of the damage caused by the sun's ultraviolet light, air pollution, and the free radicals produced in the skin as a natural byproduct of metabolism. Among the best preparations you can use on your skin are sunscreens. (For more information on these products and how they work, see chapters 10 and 12).

Even some over-the-counter preparations can have a small, but noticeable effect on the deeper layers of skin. To find out what they are and how they work—and how to be sure you're getting a product that is effective—check out chapter 10.

Asian Skin
by Andrew Wong, M.D., Ph.D., Tokyo, Japan

Although Asian skin is more resistant to sun damage because of the extra melanin it carries, Asian skin still can suffer damage from free radicals, sunlight, and oxidative stress. The best treatments take lifestyle into account and focus on antioxidants, nutritional support, and nonsurgical anti-aging treatments.

The main problem with Asian skin is that any type of inflammation (including chemical irritation, mild trauma, laser procedures, and other irritants) can lead to discoloration. Many cosmetic procedures, especially those performed by inexperienced hands, can leave unsightly blemishes due to uneven pigmentation. Sometimes the skin discoloration is so bad that we have to do corrective tattoos. I have been unable to find a laser machine that will restore natural skin color.

For maintaining a smooth and vibrant complexion, I recommend a healthy diet that hydrates the skin. I always advise Asians to drink a minimum of eight to ten glasses of water per day, and to eat plenty of antioxidant-rich fruits and vegetables. In addition, I use antioxidants like CoQ10, vitamins C and E, Beta Glucan, and lycopene, along with some herbal preparations, such as pearl powder, green tea extract, and aloe vera. Most Asians in the Far East don't worship the sun the way Americans do, but I still recommend sun protection.

Many of the procedures available in America and Europe are also used in the Far East, but microdermabrasion, lasers, and chemical peeling are less popular because of the danger of causing uneven pigmentation. Because of the increased numbers of patients requesting safe lunchtime procedures, we have begun using intense pulsed light (IPL) which uses intense broad-spectrum light to stimulate the formation of collagen and improve the skin's texture, with few side effects and very limited downtime. (For more information on IPL, see chapter 6.)

Other procedures that are effective with Asian skin include Botox injections to relax wrinkles (see chapter 4 for more information), and acupuncture (see page 61 for more information).

Australian Skin
by Joseph Georghy, M.D., Sydney, Australia

Many Australians of Northern European descent suffer from sun damage, including wrinkles, fine lines, brown and red spots, overall redness, and other skin problems. These problems are caused by exposure to Australia's intense southern sunlight, unfortunately even more so now, due to the infamous ozone hole. Many of these people have noticeably red faces, to the extent that there is a psychological condition, erythrophobia, describing their fear of their face becoming red in public.

We advise topical and physical sun protection as much as it is possible in a country where many people enjoy the outdoors. We also advise beginning rejuvenating treatments early, before the damage becomes too severe. (For more on treating this sort of skin, see chapter 8.)

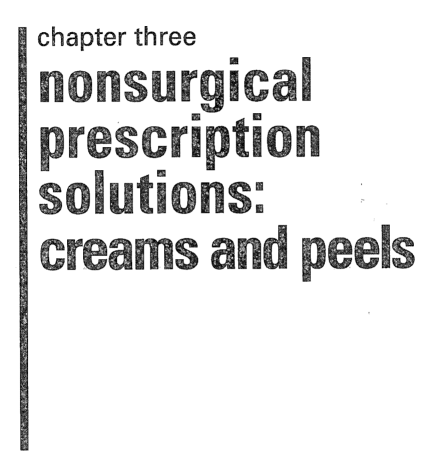

chapter three

nonsurgical prescription solutions: creams and peels

I n this chapter, we'll take a look at the latest prescription creams, lotions, peels, and masks that not only promise, but can actually restore a smooth, soft, unblemished skin to those who had given up all hope of ever looking youthful again.

wrinkles and other results of seasons in the sun

The first signs of aging that show on the skin are small wrinkles and spots or blotches, followed by furrows and sags. The age at which these unsightly blemishes start to appear is somewhat different for everyone, depending on heredity and lifestyle. You may notice such changes by your late twenties, or you could get through your forties before your skin starts to exhibit visible wear and tear. At whatever age they first appear, however, you don't have to make the inevitable signs of age a permanent part of your life.

There are more types of therapy available for facial wrinkles than for any of the other signs of aging. No wonder—these very visible folds and lines proclaim our age loud and clear.

The basic cause of a wrinkle is the breakdown of collagen and elastin. When you are young, your skin is very much like a piece of spandex—stretch it, and it snaps back into its original shape. As the spandex gets older and more worn, however, the spandex fibers stretch out and lose much of their elasticity. When you stretch the material, it may not snap back as well as it once did.

The same thing happens to your skin. As the structural and elastic fibers become old and worn, your skin becomes loose and inelastic. When it folds—as it does when you make most facial expressions—the folds tend to remain, creating those permanent creases and lines that we know as wrinkles (and that doctors call *rhytides*).

Compounding the problem of lax skin is the loss of subcutaneous fat, the layer of padding beneath the outer layer of skin. You may have noticed that older people who are overweight tend to have smoother, less lined faces than their thinner counterparts. This is partly because the layer of fat beneath their skin helps keep the skin somewhat stretched out, minimizing the appearance of wrinkles. Likewise, when you're young, your natural fat padding helps minimize the appearance of any developing lines. Once the natural fat starts to disappear, however, your wrinkles become more apparent.

You may begin to develop wrinkles as early as your late teens, depending on your skin type, genetics, and lifestyle. Those who worship the sun (and make no mistake, tanning booths also count—a lot!) or smoke invite more wrinkles earlier in life. If you tend to be very animated—if you smile and frown a lot—you're likely to develop more wrinkles more quickly than your calmer, more mysterious friends who don't let their feelings show on their faces.

Because many wrinkles, and nearly all age spots, are caused by or made worse by exposure to the sun, erstwhile beach bunnies and ski bums tend to look older than their sedentary friends. While prevention is best, modern technology can now restore the skin of even the most dedicated sun worshipper to the appearance of a Buddhist monk who's spent all of his life living in a cave.

THE TWO TYPES OF WRINKLES

There are two types of wrinkles: *dynamic*, or muscle wrinkles, that form where muscles move the face the most (around and between the eyes, and around the mouth), and *static* wrinkles, those crinkles that appear at the corners of the eyes and in other areas on the face. Because these wrinkles have very different causes, they require different treatments.

Dynamic wrinkles go deep. As they develop, they create actual furrows in the skin, like ditches in a landscape. Their appearance is obvious even when you're not moving a muscle in your face. (These permanent hyperactive lines can in turn cause static lines in the skin.) The only safe and natural-looking way to fully erase a dynamic wrinkle is to literally fill it in, though relaxing the muscles that cause the wrinkle can have a dramatic effect, as we will see in the section on Botox. (For filling in wrinkles, see chapter 5; for the use of Botox, see chapter 4.)

Static wrinkles are more superficial than dynamic wrinkles, and tend to appear most obviously when the face is moving, as when you smile or frown. These are the fine lines and crinkles, usually around the eyes, cheeks, and mouth, that can give your age away even if the rest of your face is smooth. There are a number of approaches to help minimize or eliminate these wrinkles; among them are tightening and resurfacing the skin, and eliminating unnecessary movement of the facial muscles, which will be discussed in the next chapter.

Blemishes and spots are also relatively superficial, and they too respond well to resurfacing techniques. As an added bonus, many resurfacing procedures will also help eliminate pre-cancerous skin lesions. These discolorations also respond well to various treatments with lasers and Intense Pulsed Light. (For details, see chapter 6.)

In the following pages, we will introduce you to some of the prescription products we recommend for wrinkle and blemish control.

prescription creams that can literally rejuvenate your skin

Unlike the creams and potions of years gone by that promised younger-looking skin while delivering mainly grease and moisturizer, new, cutting-edge prescription preparations actually work to rejuvenate the skin. These products are able to penetrate the outer layers of your epidermis and work from the inside, actually creating new, younger-acting, and younger-looking skin.

RETIN-A CREAMS

These products, the best known of which is the prescription cream Renova, are derived from tretinoin, a natural substance that is similar to vitamin A. It was developed originally to treat severe acne, but early researchers noticed that in addition to zapping pimples, Retin-A made the skin smoother, clearer, and firmer.

Katya, a fifty-five-year-old anthropology professor from Phoenix, mentioned that she hated the age spots that had begun to appear on her forehead and cheeks. Luckily for Katya—and for you, if you share this problem—a blotchy, uneven skin tone is one of the easiest problems to fix, and it has several possible solutions. The blotches that so bothered her were caused by too many seasons in the sun spent on archaeological digs in her case, even though she always "wore a big hat and sunscreen."

Those dreaded brown spots, referred to as "age spots" or "liver spots" (and technically as seborrheic keratoses), occur when the skin, trying to protect itself from too many ultraviolet rays, releases melanin (the dark pigment that protects the skin) unevenly. In the bad old days, people sometimes used harsh bleaching agents to fade the spots, but today there are many other options.

Katya had already let us know that she wasn't interested in any sort of medical procedure to improve her looks, but luckily she didn't need one. Instead, we prescribed Renova, a cream that helps to restore the skin's original color and texture.

"It took about three months, but it really made a difference," Katya reported later. "The splotches are mostly gone, my whole face is clearer, and my pores seem to have become smaller too."

The active ingredient in Renova, tretinoin, not only restores a youthful appearance even to sun-damaged skin, it actually repairs the sun damage. In fact, it was the first product approved by the FDA to treat sun-damaged skin.

28

How it works. Renova affects the skin on all levels. First, it speeds up the rate of cell division, causing the top layers of the skin to become thicker and smoother at the same time. The new cells actually look younger under a microscope. It also affects the melanocytes, the pigment-producing cells that cause dark spots on the skin, inducing the dark pigment to disperse more evenly and the spots to fade. There is also evidence that Renova can normalize some precancerous skin cells.

In the deeper layers of the skin, Renova increases the number of blood vessels, improving nourishment to the skin. It helps clean out and shrink deep pores, and stimulates the growth of new elastin and collagen, the skin's structural materials. Over time, the appearance of skin treated with Renova continues to improve.

How often it needs to be done. Your own doctor will put you on the best schedule for you, usually from three to seven days a week, before going to bed. Because the Retin-A molecule is unstable, you should not apply any other products to your face on the nights you use Renova, or it may not work.

How to use it. First, wash your face with a mild non-soap cleanser (such as Cetaphil, available at your local pharmacy). Pat your skin dry with a towel and let it continue to dry for ten to fifteen minutes before applying Renova. Then, apply one-pea size drop to the face each night before bed—believe it or not, this tiny amount is enough to cover your entire face. Using more will not make you look younger, faster, but is likely to lead to flaking and redness.

Renova is a cream-based product, and feels like any other facial cream going on. However, because the active ingredient causes the outer (dead) layers of the skin to slough off, other products applied to the skin penetrate more readily, which can cause stinging. (This is actually a sign that the product is working!)

Apply a moisturizer containing a sunscreen of 15 or higher to your face each morning. If the moisturizer also contains an alpha-hydroxy acid preparation, it will help the Renova work and also help counteract any dryness and scaling. Avoid sun exposure between 10 A.M. and 2 P.M. when the sun's rays are the strongest.

If your skin becomes too red and dry, decrease the application of Retin-A to every other night or even every third night.

Possible side effects and cautions. With Renova and related products, more is definitely *not better.* If you use too much or apply it too often,

Renova can cause burning, peeling, and redness. Many people find it necessary to begin gradually, using it only once or twice a week, until the skin becomes accustomed to it. This is especially important for those with very sensitive, fair skin. It also makes the skin more susceptible to the sun's rays, so a good, high-SPF (sun protection factor) sunscreen is a daily must. (See chapter 12 for a list of sunblocks and the ingredients to look for. You can also find this information on our web site in appendix B.)

People with dark skin (type IV or higher) can experience uneven pigmentation with use of Renova; if your skin is very dark, you should consider an alternative cream, such as Kinerase (see chapter 10).

If you plan to have hair removed by waxing, especially on the upper lip, stop using Renova three to four weeks prior to your treatment, or you may be left with a sore area that could heal with a brown spot. Even after you have been using Renova for several months, your skin may remain sensitive. Katya told us that during a visit to a cold and windy climate she had to reduce the number of times she applied the product, "otherwise my face got all flaky and dried out."

> **Note:** If you are pregnant, do *not* use Renova or any other product containing tretinoin, vitamin A, or retinol (an over-the-counter vitamin A preparation). Large oral doses of vitamin A have been shown to cause birth defects, and while that possibility is remote for topical applications, it is still a concern that should *not* be risked. If you are currently using Renova and are trying to conceive, discontinue it.

How long until results are apparent. It will take a few weeks to see any changes, but your skin should look younger and healthier within three months. Several studies have shown that with nightly application of Renova, the optimum results appear from six months to two years. Afterward, the product only needs to be applied one or two times a week to maintain the improvement.

Cost range. One tube of Renova lasts from three to six months, and generally costs around $55 to $65. Insurance may pay part or all of the cost if your doctor prescribes the cream for a precancerous condition.

Other prescription creams in the tretinoin family include Retin-A, used mainly for acne, and Avina, which is similar to Renova.

If you don't want to use a prescription cream, a number of over-the-counter products containing alpha-hydroxy acids or Retinol, a precursor to Retin-A, can also make a big difference in your skin's appearance, though not so dramatically nor so quickly as Renova. (See chapter 10 for more details.)

Many of our patients with splotchy skin similar to Katya's opt for a light chemical peel and/or microdermabrasion, very simple and virtually painless procedures. These and other treatments will be discussed in the next chapter.

ALPHA-HYDROXY CREAMS

Alpha-hydroxy acids, which are natural acids from such sources as apples, olives, sugar cane, and milk, have been used to beautify skin since the days of Cleopatra (remember the milk bath?). Basically, what these acids do is hasten the removal of the outer, drab, wrinkled layers of skin, producing a smoother, less blemished surface. There are literally hundreds of preparations using these natural acids, ranging from gentle lotions you can apply at home (for details, see chapter 10) to prescription-strength creams and lotions you can obtain from your doctor.

One of the most effective forms of alpha-hydroxy acid is glycolic acid, derived primarily from sugar cane. Glycolic acid creams and lotions can be applied at night, before you go to bed, and again in the morning before you apply your sunscreen. They can also be used in conjunction with Renova and Kinerase, an over-the-counter rejuvenating product, though not at the same time. We suggest Renova be applied three to five nights per week, then use a prescribed glycolic acid product the remaining nights. The two types of products seem to enhance one another's effects.

light peels (prescription strength)

Natural acid peels are another time-honored way to freshen and rejuvenate the appearance of aging skin. These can range from very light peels that can be applied at home to prescription-strength light and medium peels applied in a medical setting. Deep peels, which we do not recommend because they damage the deepest layers of the skin, should only be applied by a doctor. They also carry a small risk of infection, scarring, and skin discoloration. While the skin will eventually heal, resulting in a younger-looking complexion, the process is potentially very damaging and doesn't always yield the smooth-looking results you want.

More superficial peels, which we do recommend, generally make use of glycolic acid (an alpha-hydroxy acid) to gently remove the top layers of the skin without irritation, burning, or drying, revealing the smoother, more youthful-looking skin beneath.

Bear in mind that peels can be applied to your whole face, or to a specific area, such as the forehead, cheeks, or around the mouth.

ALPHA PEELS (GLYCOLIC ACID, ALPHA HYDROXY ACID)

You've probably heard of the "lunchtime peel," so-called because it can be done quickly and has few side effects. These peels, which must be done by your doctor, usually use a 35 to 50 percent solution of glycolic acid, and can be applied to both the face and neck. Alpha peels are usually administered once a week for two to six weeks. In addition to exfoliating the outermost layers of dead skin cells, thus removing the gray or lifeless-looking superficial layers of skin, these peels also speed the renewal of those top layers. In the proper strength, they can diminish or remove spots, as well as increase collagen production, helping to restore the skin's firmness and elasticity.

Before having an alpha peel, be sure to follow the general cautions detailed below. Note that if you have darker skin color, alpha peels can cause an increase in melanin, which can lead to a blotchy look.

BETA PEELS(SALICYLIC ACID)

Beta-hydroxy acids, of which salicylic acid is the most often used, are believed to be comparable in their effects to alpha-hydroxy acids, but are less irritating to the skin and may be more appropriate for people with dark complexions, in whom they are less likely to cause an increase in skin pigmentation.

What to do before. For a week before having any sort of peel, it's important to discontinue the use of Renova or any other product containing tretinoin, as well as depilatories, home facial masks, exfoliating sponges, or loofahs. You should also avoid shaving facial hair or getting electrolysis treatments. Your doctor may prescribe a preparatory cream or lotion to use in the week before the peel, although on the day of the peel itself you should use nothing on your face.

You should never have a peel if you have an active outbreak of herpes, a severe sunburn, any abrasions or scratches on your face, or if you have recently received radiation treatments.

If you easily scar, or you have a connective tissue disorder, such as lupus, you should avoid any sort of peels. If you have a history of allergies, you should have your doctor or cosmetician apply a patch test before proceeding with a general peel. If you have dark skin, discuss possible side effects with your doctor; even light peels can cause uneven pigmentation on brown and black skin.

On the day of the peel, do not shave or apply any sort of preparation to your face.

The procedure. When you have a superficial peel, the doctor may first apply a numbing cream to your skin, then gently apply the alpha solution to your whole face or a part of it. You will probably feel a tingling or even a mild burning or stinging sensation as the compound begins to work. Be sure to let your doctor know what you are feeling. When the peel is done, the doctor or aesthetician may apply a neutralizing solution and then will wash all traces of the acid off your face, often followed by the application of a soothing lotion.

How long it takes. Generally, the doctor will leave the peel on your face for two to five minutes. The strength of the preparation and the amount of time it is left on may gradually be increased with subsequent treatments.

How often it needs to be done. An initial treatment is usually done once a week for two to six weeks. Because superficial peels are relatively mild, they can be repeated whenever you feel the need for a beauty boost. Many of our clients prefer the immediate effects of microdermabrasion. (See page 34.)

What to do after. The immediate effect of a superficial peel is similar to that of a mild sunburn. Expect some redness and peeling for up to three to five days. Your doctor will probably prescribe a cream to soothe your skin, which you should apply as directed. Your doctor may advise you not to apply make-up for a few hours after the peel. In addition, you should avoid using any alpha-hydroxy or tretinoin products (such as Renova) for at least 48 hours. Avoid the sun as much as possible and be sure to wear a good sunscreen whenever you go into the sun, both immediately after the peel and forever afterward. This is a good idea for everyone anyway.

Possible side effects and cautions. The long-term effects of using alpha hydroxy and beta peels are unknown. In the short term, these peels can irritate the skin, especially alpha peels. In rare cases, the skin can swell and blister. If you notice excessive redness and burning after your treatment, you may be oversensitive to the ingredients in the peel, and should consider a different formulation or a different method of rejuvenating your skin.

How long till results are apparent. Although your skin will probably be pink right after the peel, this should fade within a few hours to a few days. Apart from this slight reddening, you should notice a smoother and clearer-looking complexion after the first treatment, which will improve even more as the treatments continue.

Cost range. Each alpha peel generally costs from $60 to $100, depending on the part of the country where you have it done. With multiple peels, the cost per peel may be reduced. The costs for beta peels are comparable.

microdermabrasion

Alyssa, age thirty, is a supermodel whose face has graced the covers of the top fashion magazines. This tall Dutch beauty has honey-colored hair and flawless, glowing skin. But her skin wasn't flawless when she first came to see us. Her skin was discolored and bumpy, and, she says, "People were always telling me I looked tired."

Though a natural beauty, Alyssa was beginning to show the normal skin signs of aging. Not a problem for most of us in our early thirties—but thirty is considered old for a model. Alyssa feared that her less-than-perfect complexion might prevent her continuing in her profession.

We recommended a number of treatments, including immediate microdermabrasion to smooth her skin and get rid of the small imperfections. Alyssa says, "At first it stung, and I couldn't see a difference. But after the third treatment, people started asking me if I'd gone on holiday. 'Your skin looks so good,' they said."

After two months of biweekly treatments, the difference in Alyssa's face was dramatic. She said, "My face looks better than it ever has. A few weeks after I started the treatments, I got a contract with Ford [one of the biggest international modeling agencies]," she added proudly. "I'd also had my hair cut shorter, and I know luck always plays a big part, but maybe it was also because of the treatments."

Microdermabrasion is one of the quickest and easiest ways to improve any less-than-perfect complexion. Although it will do nothing for deep wrinkles, microdermabrasion removes all surface imperfections, including blackheads, age spots, discolorations, fine wrinkles, and lines. Your pores will appear smaller and your skin may appear to glow, as if you had just received a facial.

Because microdermabrasion is so gentle, it can be performed as often as weekly, and the results just keep getting better.

How it works. Microdermabrasion, jokingly called "sandblasting" by some of our clients, uses a special machine that sprays a fine mist of microscopic crystals (most commonly aluminum oxide, sometimes sodium hydroxide) onto your skin, then immediately vacuums them up again, along with the dead skin cells scrubbed off by the crystals. This is actually a form of very superficial peel, targeting only the outermost layers of the skin. No anesthetic is required, and you can return to your regular activities immediately afterward. Microdermabrasion is performed in some beauty spas, but spas are limited in the power of the machines that they are permitted to use, so their peels will be more superficial than those performed in a doctor's office.

What to do before. As with any medical procedure, you'll need to meet with your doctor to discuss your general health and any medications you are taking beforehand. Those who should *not* receive microdermabrasion include skin cancer patients, diabetics, anyone with open sores of any sort, including herpes, and anyone who has undergone facial or neck surgery of any sort within the previous three months. If you are currently using Accutane, you must discontinue it for six months before treatment because it can increase the chances of scarring.

> **Note:** There are a number of microdermabrasion machines available. Make sure that your doctor or aesthetician uses a reputable one, such as Dermapeel, Power Peel, Smart Peel, Parisian Peel, and Mega-Peel. Don't be afraid to ask about the type of machine when you make your appointment. The best machines make use of a closed system in which the crystals are discarded once used and are never reused. Avoid going to practitioners who reuse the crystals. They are not meant to be reused.

The procedure. For most people, the sensation of having microdermabrasion is like being in a strong wind. Some report a slight stinging, especially around the eyes. While the treatment is being done, you will hear a gentle hum as the machine vacuums away your old, dead skin cells.

Afterward, you may feel as if you have received a mild sun- or windburn. Any pinkness or minor discomfort should disappear completely within a few hours.

How long it takes. An average full-face treatment should take about half an hour. If you have your neck and upper chest done as well, it will take longer, up to an hour.

How often it needs to be done. We recommend an initial series of four to eight treatments spaced ten days to two weeks apart. Afterward, you will need a touchup procedure once every two or three months to keep your skin looking its best. The strength of the crystal spray may be gradually increased over the course of your treatment cycle.

What to do after. After the treatment, the doctor will give you a soothing lotion, which you should apply as directed. Stay out of direct sunlight as much as possible for several days, and always wear an SPF 15 or higher sunscreen. Avoid using any Retin-A, alpha-hydroxy, or glycolic acid product for at least 72 hours after receiving microdermabrasion.

Possible side effects and cautions. Microdermabrasion is safe and effective for most skin types. You should probably not have this treatment, however, if you are prone to developing keloids. Other side effects that can occasionally occur include outbreaks of herpes; eye irritation caused by the microcrystals used in the process (rinsing your eye with an eyewash should alleviate any discomfort); redness, which should subside in a few hours; increased sensitivity to the sun; and bleeding, which is very rare. You should also be aware that microdermabrasion can occasionally cause areas of uneven pigmentation on brown and black skin.

How long until results are apparent. You should see an improvement in your skin's texture and clarity by the second or third treatment. Your complexion will improve even more with each subsequent "sandblasting." Many people report that their skin has *never* looked so good, not even when they were very young.

Cost range. A single treatment costs between $75 and $200, depending on where you live and where you have the procedure done. The national average is around $135. Check to see if there is a discount for a series of treatments.

microcurrent nonsurgical "facelift"

Microcurrent technology, which makes use of tiny amounts of electrical current to stimulate body tissues, has been used for more than 20 years in the medical field to treat Bell's Palsy and other forms of facial paralysis. Recently, especially in Europe, it is also used to improve some of the signs of aging, such as wrinkling and sagging, by stimulating and toning the facial muscles and speeding up the regeneration of skin tissue. It is also used to facilitate lymphatic drainage, which can reduce the appearance of puffiness under the eyes.

How it works. The current that comes from the socket in your home that powers your lamps, television and other devices, is measured in "amps." The microcurrent used to rejuvenate your skin is measured in "microamps"—each of which is one one-millionth of an amp. This small amount of current is insufficient to stimulate muscle movement, or even be felt, but strong enough to lead to rejuvenating effects.

In addition to stimulating cell regeneration, microcurrent causes constriction of blood vessels, which can lead to a reduction in redness of the skin in such conditions as rosacea.

What to do before. Before your procedure, you should tell your doctor about the medications you are taking. If you have certain medical conditions, your doctor needs to know, as there is a mild possibility they could be affected by the small amount of current used. These conditions include epilepsy, diabetes, pregnancy, having a metal plate in your head, or having a cardiac pacemaker.

The Procedure. There is no preparation involved before your microcurrent procedure. You will be seated in a comfortable medical chair, and the doctor will apply probes to the areas to be treated. Depending on the machine used and the areas to be treated, you may feel a mild tingling sensation during the procedure. Most people feel nothing at all.

from 15 to 60 minutes. Many people find the treatments relaxing; in fact, it is common for some patients to fall asleep during treatments.

While there are many machines available we prefer to use the "Perfector" which has the best tailored programs for all skin types.

chapter four
muscle relaxing injections

When your grandmother or next-door neighbor had plastic surgery thirty years ago—or your coworker had a deep peel last summer—chances are you were told that she had gone away on vacation for a few weeks. This was because of the time it took to heal from these procedures which were, in the first case, serious surgery, and in the second, a procedure akin to having the facial skin burned off. Healing involved pain and other discomfort, as well as a much worse-looking appearance for a few weeks to many months.

When the person who had undergone these rejuvenating treatments returned, he or she probably looked better—more rested and younger—but may also have looked odd. After surgery, it's not uncommon for the face to become somewhat asymmetrical and the skin discolored, from the disrupted blood supply. Or perhaps this person's skin retained a "shiny," healing appearance, even many weeks or months after the peel or surgery. Although both of these procedures can eventually produce good results, they are extreme measures, not to mention very costly.

Today there are a number of new medical (but nonsurgical) procedures that can offer you that rested-looking, youthful appearance immediately, without any downtime, and no recovery period. All these new procedures, which are widely available all over the country, are becoming less expensive all the time.

Perhaps the best known of the miraculous new youth-promoting treatments is Botox. In our opinion, Botox is a true modern miracle: a deadly poison that has been tamed to erase or ease worry lines, forehead wrinkles, crows' feet, lines around and above the mouth, neck folds, and even excessive sweating (hyperhidrosis). (Botox is also useful in a wide variety of medical conditions that had no previous treatment.) Currently, and probably for some time to come, Botox treatments are the most widely performed of all cosmetic procedures in the United States.

HOW IT WORKS

Botox was developed for medical use from the toxin of the bacterium *Clostridium botulinum*, which causes a particularly deadly form of food poisoning, botulism. The reason botulism can be so deadly is that it causes widespread paralysis of all the body's muscles and without treatment can result in death by suffocation.

How could something so lethal become so useful to modern medicine? The answer is that scientists found a way to purify the toxin and apply it in miniscule amounts to target specific muscles. Botox, manufactured by Allergan, was first used widely to treat uncontrolled eye spasms. It was approved for this use in the late 1980s by the Food and Drug Administration. Botox was so successful that doctors began using it off-label for a variety of other conditions caused by muscle spasms. Eye doctors using it for eye spasms noticed that their patients began looking younger and more relaxed because the muscles that caused squint and frown lines were also relaxed.

Throughout the 1990s, dermatologists, plastic surgeons, and other physicians began using Botox to treat a growing number of cosmetic imperfections caused by overactive muscles. Unlike injectable fillers, which fill in the skin underneath a wrinkle, or CoolTouch laser treatments, which create new collagen under the wrinkle, Botox actually goes to the source of dynamic wrinkles by preventing the excessive muscular activity in the first place.

To picture how it works, imagine that your skin is a bed sheet with two people pulling on opposite corners, creating a diagonal furrow. Then, if both people drop the sheet, you can smooth it out, eliminating the furrow and associat-

muscle relaxing injections

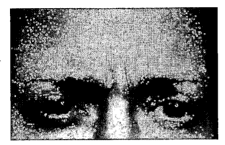
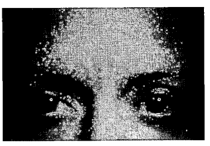

Pre Botox: Glabella frowning   After Botox: Glabella frowning

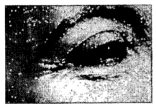
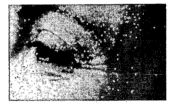

Pretreatment: Crows feet, smiling

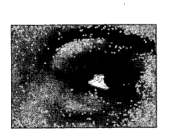
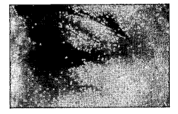

Two weeks after Botox, smiling

ed wrinkles. That's something like what happens with Botox. A minute amount of poison is injected into or around a muscle, where it is absorbed by the nerve that tells the muscle to contract through a chemical signal. Botox prevents the nerve from communicating with the muscle, thus weakening it or paralyzing it. This allows the affected muscle to relax and in turn lets the skin smooth out over the facial structure.

In early 2002, Allergan obtained approval by the FDA for Botox as a cosmetic treatment for frown lines between the eyebrows; other cosmetic uses are therefore still off-label. However, off-label use is a common and usually very safe practice with many drugs.

Botox is most effective in the forehead and eye areas, erasing furrows between the brows, vertical lines in the forehead, squint lines around the eyes (crow's feet), and lines under the eyes or on the sides of the nose. The affected muscles will have greatly decreased motion; if too much Botox is injected, however, they will not move at all and the face will be lacking in expression. It's important to choose a doctor with the experience and intelligence to inject exactly the right amount of Botox for your particular situation.

Because the muscles that surround the mouth are so important to so many functions—talking, eating, smiling, kissing—we use Botox only sparingly and very carefully in this area. Still, doctors are increasingly using Botox injections to improve the appearance of lines around the mouth (nasolabial folds) or from the mouth to the chin (marionette lines), as well as the small vertical lines that often appear above the mouth (lipstick lines). While Botox alone can't completely eliminate those lines, it can make a big difference.

For the best results—virtual elimination of all lines around the mouth—it's best to combine Botox with injectable implants, which can fill in the ugly lines. Botox, by relaxing the responsible muscles, keeps the implants in place and helps prevent the lines from reforming. CoolTouch laser treatments are also very helpful in this area.

One of the most exciting recent uses of Botox is in improving the appearance of an aging neck. We use Botox in two ways for this purpose, both involving the platysma muscles, which lie very close to the surface of the neck. With age, the platysma muscles can sag, causing tell-tale horizontal lines in the front of the neck. In many people, they also separate into strings, causing the gaunt, ugly "turkey neck" effect. When the platysma muscles are treated with Botox, however, they relax, their stringiness disappears, and the neck begins to resume a younger appearance.

The best thing about using Botox to erase facial or neck wrinkles, besides

muscle relaxing injections

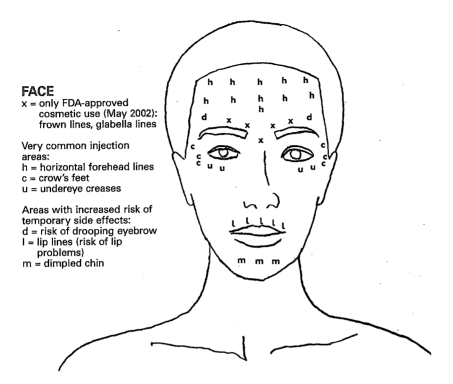

FACE
x = only FDA-approved
    cosmetic use (May 2002):
    frown lines, glabella lines

Very common injection
areas:
h = horizontal forehead lines
c = crow's feet
u = undereye creases

Areas with increased risk of
temporary side effects:
d = risk of drooping eyebrow
l = lip lines (risk of lip
    problems)
m = dimpled chin

its great results, is that it doesn't affect any muscles other than those that are targeted. You will still be able to smile, laugh, and even show displeasure, but without the wrinkle-producing side-effects.

WHAT TO DO BEFORE

We believe that the best outcomes result from good communication between doctors and patients. Be sure to discuss any concerns you have with your doctor before the procedure, and discuss any medical conditions and medications you are taking that might affect the successful outcome. In particular, we recommend letting your doctor know about any allergies you may have, including food and drug allergies or allergies to environmental elements.

In addition to the list of all medications and supplements you are currently taking, it's also important to give your doctor the names of all the vitamins, herbs, and over-the-counter remedies you also take. This is because some anti-inflammatory medications, including aspirin, may lead to increased bruising from Botox injections. Vitamin E can also slightly increase the risk of bruising. Some antibiotics and other medicines can actually increase the potency of Botox, which means that you would need a smaller dose.

During your initial meeting or just before your procedure, you will be asked to sign an informed consent release, stating that you have been informed about all possible complications of Botox injections.

THE PROCEDURE

You will be seated upright in a medical chair. Your doctor may apply ice to the affected site, both to dull the very minor pain of injection and to prevent bleeding or bruising. The doctor will then ask you to strongly contract the muscle that is responsible for the wrinkle she is treating, so she can pinpoint the exact site for the injections.

- For forehead lines, raise your eyebrows
- For crow's feet, smile or squint
- For furrows between the eyebrows, frown
- For lines beneath the eyes, squint
- For lipstick lines, purse your lips
- For nasolabial folds and marionette lines, smile
- For chin wrinkles, purse your lips
- For neck lines or turkey neck, grimace

Once the doctor has determined exactly where to position the needle, she will administer the injections. The average number of injections per site is three. You will feel a needle prick from the tiny microneedle at the site of each injection, and then a mild stinging for a few seconds as the toxin is injected. The whole process takes from about ten minutes to half an hour, depending on the number of areas being treated. As soon as the procedure is completed, you can return to your normal activities.

HOW OFTEN IT NEEDS TO BE DONE

One injection generally lasts three to six months, though in some cases it can last up to a year. The amount of time a treatment lasts largely depends on the site of the injection. As the toxin wears off, the wrinkles will gradually return, but they won't be any worse than before the treatment. With repeated injections, each treatment tends to last longer. There is some evidence that after prolonged treatment, the muscles affected permanently lose their tone, so only occasional further treatments will be needed, if at all.

One of our patients, who was a Botox pioneer—she's been receiving treatments for over ten years—tells us that the last time she received Botox for the furrows between her eyebrows was over two years ago. "I just haven't needed it," she said happily.

WHAT TO DO AFTER

Your doctor may ask you to hold an ice pack to the site of the injections for a few minutes after the injections, especially if you were treated in the area around the eye, which has very thin skin and bruises easily. To prevent the injected toxin from spreading to adjacent muscles, you will also be asked not to rub the area, and not to bend over or lie down for several hours.

POSSIBLE SIDE EFFECTS AND CAUTIONS

Botox causes few side effects. You may have a small bruise at the site of the injection that will fade in a few days. In rare cases, Botox injections around the eye area can cause your eyelid to droop, though this will wear off in two or three weeks. It is even rarer, but possible, for injections in the neck muscles to cause difficulty with swallowing. This too will wear off in a short period of time. Be sure to discuss all these possibilities with your doctor before beginning treatment and to let her know if any of these side effects appear.

One of the few drawbacks to using Botox is that some people develop a resistance to it after repeated injections, and it no longer works. Luckily for these patients, scientists are working on producing alternative drugs based on other forms of the botulinum toxin (Botox is made from botulinum type A).

One of these new drugs, Myobloc, manufactured by Elan Pharmaceuticals, based on botulinum type B, is already FDA approved (cosmetic use is off-label) and on the market as an alternative to Botox. Myobloc works well for those who have developed resistance to Botox. It is also much easier for physicians to work with because it comes pre-mixed and has a long shelf life of more than a year in the refrigerator. Botox must be mixed with sterile, preservative-free saline just before use, and lasts only a day or two in the refrigerator.

The jury is still out, but for cosmetic use, Myobloc lasts two to four months compated with Botox, which lasts three to six months before another treatment is needed. This seems to depend upon the exact procedure, but the onset of Myobloc's effect is quicker, and in all other respects it produces nearly identical results to those of Botox.

Researchers are working on creating drugs from the five other types of botulinum toxin. It is likely that several of them will be developed in the future for even more medical uses, and bioengineered toxins may eventually be developed as well.

HOW LONG UNTIL RESULTS ARE APPARENT

It generally takes three to seven days to see maximum results from a Botox treatment. If, after a week, you feel there has been no improvement, consult your doctor, who may perform a touch-up Botox treatment or may use another type of botulinum toxin.

COST RANGE

The cost of Botox treatments depends on your geographical location and where you go for treatment, as well as the part of your face you want treated. Most doctors charge by the site, meaning the area in which you are injected, although others charge by the injection. The area between the eyebrows (glabella) is considered one site, the forehead is one site, the crow's feet on either side are together considered one site, and the regions below the eyes might also be considered a separate site.

In general, forehead injections are more expensive than those for crows' feet because they require more of the toxin. Treatment of the neck is more costly still. Count on a per treatment range of between $300 and $2000 ($300 to $500 per site). It is common practice to reduce the charge when more than one site is done at the same session.

Why are Botox treatments so costly? Botox is an expensive drug; it costs more than $400 for a vial that will treat one to four people, depending upon the areas treated, and of course there are other costs involved. Once mixed, Botox loses effectiveness with time, and is best used the day it is prepared or within a day or two at most. Your doctor will usually try to schedule two or more patients on the same day in order to use the Botox efficiently. If your charge is much less than the range mentioned above, it is possible that the Botox has been over-diluted or it is older and might be less effective.

Remember, too, that you are also paying for your doctor's experience. According to Dr. Malcolm Paul of the American Society for Aesthetic Plastic Surgery, "People may think that the procedure is only a simple injection and not realize that it requires an in-depth knowledge of the facial muscles and the relationship of these

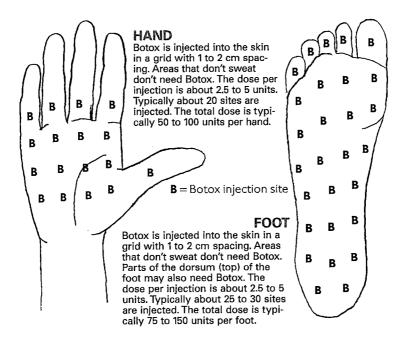

HAND
Botox is injected into the skin in a grid with 1 to 2 cm spacing. Areas that don't sweat don't need Botox. The dose per injection is about 2.5 to 5 units. Typically about 20 sites are injected. The total dose is typically 50 to 100 units per hand.

B = Botox injection site

FOOT
Botox is injected into the skin in a grid with 1 to 2 cm spacing. Areas that don't sweat don't need Botox. Parts of the dorsum (top) of the foot may also need Botox. The dose per injection is about 2.5 to 5 units. Typically about 25 to 30 sites are injected. The total dose is typically 75 to 150 units per foot.

muscles to normal facial movement." This is why it's essential to choose a board-certified physician with appropriate training and experience.

hyperhidrosis (excessive sweating)

Although not strictly a cosmetic problem, hyperhidrosis, or excessive sweating, has long been a problem for many people in the public eye as well as in private life. In the 1987 movie *Broadcast News*, Albert Brooks plays an aspiring newscaster who sweats so badly from the forehead that a few minutes into the newscast, small rivers of perspiration are seen running down his face.

Although Brooks's problem was overplayed for comic effect in that movie, those who suffer from hyperhidrosis often perspire so heavily that their clothing and even shoes (if the problem is on the soles of their feet) can quickly be ruined. Those with sweaty palms are reluctant to shake hands and often have to wear gloves to absorb the excess sweat.

Until Botox, the options for people with this unfortunate condition were limited: antiperspirants, which were usually useless; systemic drugs, which were of limited effectiveness and sometimes had serious side effects; excision of the sweat glands, a drastic remedy; and sympathectomy, or cutting the sympathetic nerves to the affected area or areas. The sympathetic nerves, part of the autonomic nervous system, govern many of our body's automatic activities, such as digestion and sweating. Sympathectomy is another drastic remedy, and while it sometimes gives gratifying results, it often fails or results in "paradoxical," or rebound sweating from other areas. The good news is that Botox can inactivate these nerves, just like the nerves to our voluntary muscles. After injections of Botox, the sweat glands no longer receive the message to produce perspiration, thus drying up the problem for several months to more than a year.

In one case, a law student who had suffered from hyperhidrosis for years was able to resume a normal life; in another, a man who had seemingly incurable warts on his feet was completely cured when we stopped the excessive sweating that had provided a welcoming environment for the warts.

When used for weakening overactive muscles, Botox is injected into the muscle. For hyperhidrosis, Botox is injected into the skin of the area that produces excessive perspiration, avoiding the muscle. This is more painful and sometimes has a side effect of temporary and very slight weakness in the adjacent muscles.

For excessive sweating in the forehead, a number of very small, closely spaced injections of Botox are given throughout the area of greatest perspiration. Cosmetic Botox injections can decrease forehead sweating as a bonus.

In the armpit area, the doctor will first perform a test to determine the areas of greatest perspiration, then inject small amounts of Botox throughout those areas. For most patients, no anesthetic is necessary beyond a skin-numbing cream.

Although Botox treatments significantly reduce or even eliminate the most copious armpit sweating, that from the eccrine sweat glands, it has no effect on the other type of sweat glands, the apocrine glands, which produce "nervous" sweat. As a result, armpit odor may still be a problem, but it can be more easily controlled through cleanliness and deodorants.

Because of the potential discomfort involved, we often use a regional anesthetic (a nerve block) when treating the palms of the hands or soles of the feet. Application of ice to the area or spraying with ethylchloride, a cooling and numbing spray, are often sufficient. Once the area is numb, we inject the toxin in very small, precise doses along a grid covering the palm or sole of the foot.

After being treated with Botox for hyperhidrosis, you may need to return for evaluation. In some cases, you'll need a few supplemental injections to cover any small areas that are still producing excessive perspiration. Occasionally the treatment is too effective and daily application of moisturizer is necessary.

Botox for hyperhidrosis can take more than a week to achieve its maximal benefit, so be patient and take comfort in the fact that it lasts considerably longer than many other uses of Botox; in one study the effect lasted more than ten months in half the patients who received it.

chapter five

injectable
implants

Sometimes the deep furrows between your eyes will be helped only slightly by Botox. Other deep muscle wrinkles, such as the lines around your mouth and from your mouth to your chin (marionette lines) result not only from repeated muscle movement and loss of skin tone, but also as a result of the loss of underlying fat (see "Anatomy of a Wrinkle," in chapter 3).

Although improving skin tone and texture, through exfoliating (peels, microdermabrasion) and stimulating the deep tissues to produce new collagen (CoolTouch), can improve the appearance of these prominent lines, they can only be truly erased by filling in the sunken areas beneath the skin.

For years, implants of bovine and human cadaver collagen have been used to fill in and plump out depressed areas of the skin, from deep wrinkles to scars. The problem with collagen, however, is that it is relatively short-acting, often needing to be replaced in as little as three to six weeks. Also, many people have allergic reactions to collagen of animal origin. Collagen injections can also be distributed unevenly, forming unsightly lumps and bumps.

A number of promising new implant materials have come on the market in recent years, offering a far better and longer-lasting outcome than collagen. Because most of them are inert substances, they offer little danger of allergic reactions.

two types of implants

These new implants fall into two categories: permanent and biodegradable. The permanent implants are, as advertised, permanent. Their effects can be very gratifying. While this may sound at first like the ideal solution, we usually don't recommend them because of several problems reported to have occurred with some patients.

PERMANENT FILLERS

The first problem with permanent implants is that these substances (like all implants) can migrate from the site where they were implanted, forming unsightly lumps. However, because the permanent fillers do not degrade, the lumps are permanent unless surgically removed—and in some cases not even then, if the filler material bonds with the body's own tissues. Likewise, if one of these implants is injected too superficially it will form a permanent ridge or lump that will have to be removed surgically.

A more serious problem is that in rare cases these permanent substances can cause a local inflammatory reaction called a granuloma, which can result in extensive breakdown of facial tissue and can even require reconstructive surgery.

BIODEGRADABLE FILLERS

There is a wide and growing variety of temporary and long-lasting (but not permanent) biodegradable substances used to fill in wrinkles and scars, and for other cosmetic purposes. One that you may have heard of, which has been increasingly used by many physicians, is autologous fat. This fat is taken via liposuction from some part of your body where you don't want it (abdomen, buttocks) and injected into wrinkles or facial folds. The main advantage to using the body's own fat is that there is no danger of an allergic reaction. The results also look good, but they are comparatively short-lived. For this reason, and also because this filler is more complicated to use (requiring two procedures), we don't recommend it.

Instead, we recommend (and mostly employ) biodegradable fillers. Although they aren't forever, most of them are quite long-lasting. The implants we use are made from various natural substances, including hyaluronic acid, a natural component of the skin that fills the spaces between the skin's collagen and elastin. Because of its role in natural physiological processes, hyaluronic acid has a wide and growing range of medical uses in dermatology, rheumatology, orthopedics, and ophthalmology.

Long used in Europe and Canada, the new injectable fillers can be used to fill in scars, including acne scars, as well as deep folds and wrinkles caused by muscle movement or loss of collagen, elastin, and fat. They are also used to smooth the area above the lips as well as for plumping out lip tissue itself.

Please be aware that although they are widely used in Europe and throughout the world, not all filler substances described below have been approved for cosmetic use by the FDA. *The following are recommeded fillers.*

Reviderm. In our opinion, this is one of the best of the fillers, with the least likelihood of adverse effects. Made of hyaluronic acid and microbeads of dextran, an inert medical substance, Reviderm is injected through a microneedle into the wrinkle, scar, lip, or other area to be treated.

The treated area will look better immediately, partly because of swelling, and will continue to improve as the injection stimulates new collagen to form. Eventually, the body's own collagen will encapsulate the dextran beads, leading to a natural-looking fullness that should last at least 6 months and up to a year and a half.

The hyaluronic acid in Reviderm is made by bacteria, using recombinant DNA. Because it contains no animal products, there's virtually no chance of an allergic reaction with Reviderm, so there's no need for an allergy test beforehand. The hyaluronic acid is slightly modified to make it last longer in the body. Similar hyaluronic acid products include Restylane, Hylaform, Rofilan, and Perlane. As of February 2003 none of these is FDA approved.

New-Fill (polylactic acid). This long-lasting injectable substance is a polymer of lactic acid (a naturally occurring substance) containing no animal products and with no risk of allergic reaction. When used as a filler it has a double action: first, it fills in the wrinkle or scar where it is injected; later it stimulates formation of natural collagen at the place where it has been injected. The collagen formation continues even after the polylactic acid has been absorbed by the body, and it typically lasts from a few months to a year.

A single treatment should cost between $500 and $1000. New-Fill has been used for over twenty years in Europe, but is not yet FDA approved as of February 2003.

Evolution. This is a strictly non-animal product made of the same material as surgical sutures. Once it is inserted, it serves as a scaffolding for your body's own natural collagen. Although treatment with Evolution may need to be repeated after a few weeks, the ultimate improvement is long-lasting. Not yet FDA approved.

You should consider these fillers with care:

Artecoll. This permanent filler consists of microspheres made from an inert medical material, polymethylmethacrylate (PMMA, similar to superglue and the cement used by orthopedists), suspended in a solution of bovine collagen. Generally considered safe, Artecoll has been used in Europe, Canada, and South America for over ten years.

Within a few weeks after implantation, Artecoll's microspheres (which are smaller in diameter than a human hair) become encapsulated and anchored by your body's own natural collagen. Despite its general record of safety, we seldom recommend Artecoll and other permanent fillers because of the small possibility of granuloma. Also, the bovine collagen element can provoke a rare allergic reaction. Not yet FDA approved.

Gore-Tex (for lips). This permanent (but reversible) implant is made from the same futuristic material that keeps your feet dry while hiking. The material, expanded polytetrafluoroethylene (ePTFE), has a soft, natural feel and is provided in the form of very tiny threads. It is nonreactive, and the body's own tissues eventually bond to it. Gore-Tex is most often used for lip augmentation (see chapter 8 for details). Smaller threads are sometimes used to plump out wrinkles, especially the deep creases from the nose to the chin (nasolabial folds and marionette lines). If placed imperfectly, or if the threads are too large in diameter, Gore-Tex implants can form visible or palpable lines under the skin. Similar implants include the brand names Softform and UltraSoft.

Dermalogen. This and other similar fillers is actually made from donated human tissue (from cadavers) that has been processed for purity. In addition, antiviral agents are applied to the product to make certain that no viruses are present. Dermalogen can be used like any other injectable filler, and has the advantage of never causing an allergic reaction. Essentially, Dermalogen and similar products work by creating a sort of internal scaffolding for natural collagen to grow into.

One drawback is that this filler may not be as long-lasting as some of the newer synthetic fillers. In addition, Dermalogen may require several injections over a period of two to three months to obtain optimal results. Other products that use processed human skin or fascia (the tissue that covers and binds muscles) include Cymetra, Fascian, and Alloderm.

These fillers are not recommended:

Silicone. This has been made famous (or infamous) as a breast implant material, is a filler made from a purified compound of the mineral silica and oxygen. Injected as silicone oil, the filler material consists of microdroplets of silicone which disperse through the injection site and are then surrounded by the body's own cells.

Unlike collagen, silicone is permanent and never hardens. It is also extremely inexpensive compared to other filler materials. However, when problems do arise with silicone they can be severe and even disfiguring. There are cases of implants shifting after many months or even years, forming permanent lumps in parts of the face where they are unwanted.

In addition to its tendency to shift, silicone also poses the danger of inflammation, infection, or severe allergic reaction, often long after the material was injected. Because it is a permanent filler, it is extremely difficult, if not impossible, to remove if deleterious side effects occur.

The FDA web site states: "The FDA has not approved the marketing of liquid silicone for injection for any cosmetic purpose, including the treatment of facial defects or wrinkles, or enlarging the breasts. The adverse effects of liquid silicone injections have included movement of the silicone to other parts of the body, inflammation and discoloration of surrounding tissues, and the formation of granulomas (nodules of granulated, inflamed tissue)."

The bottom line, as far as we're concerned, is to avoid any silicone-based implants, and steer clear of physicians who recommend them.

Collagen. Widely used since the 1970s, collagen is a natural product made from the skins of young calves. Because many people are allergic to bovine protein, use of this product requires a skin test from four to six weeks before the procedure (although most reactions show up within three days). Once the collagen has been injected, the doctor will massage the area of injection to make certain that it was distributed evenly. The area will be very swollen right after the injection, but should look natural within a few hours to a day.

It is about average in cost as a filler material, but the results are very short-lived, from one to six months. Also, as we mentioned before, allergic reactions to collagen are not uncommon. Well-known brand names include Zyderm and Zyplast.

Autologous fat. The advantage of using your own fat seem obvious: since the doctor is injecting your own tissue, and it is replacing your body's own fat that has been lost, there is no danger of rejection.

The disadvantages, however, outweigh the advantages in our opinion. First, this requires two procedures rather than one: the initial liposuction, which has its own risks, and then the implantation of the suctioned-out fat, after it has been processed to remove excess fluids. Second, even with careful handling, the fat cells may not survive the process. Instead of providing padding beneath your wrinkles, they will simply be absorbed into the body. There is no way to predict how much of the fat will survive. Third, the procedure is very specialized and requires a very skilled and experienced physician.

The jury is still out on how long autologous fat transplants last. Common estimates range from six months to several years, depending upon the site of the injection.

Whatever filler you and your doctor choose, the basic procedure is essentially the same (except for autologous fat implantation, which is preceded by liposuction).

HOW FILLERS WORK

All the injectables work by filling in and plumping up the depressed area beneath a scar, or wrinkle, or fold. In addition, many of them also stimulate production of the body's own natural collagen and provide a framework for it. Most fillers are also suitable for helping to fill in the narrow "smoker's lines" above the lips and for plumping up the lips themselves and returning them to the sensuous fullness of youth.

WHAT TO DO BEFORE

As with any medical procedure, you must discuss your general health with your doctor before receiving implants, including any medications you are taking. You will be advised to discontinue aspirin or any other medication that can increase bleeding (including vitamin E). Also, because the safety of implants has not been evaluated for pregnant women, tell your doctor if you are pregnant or planning to conceive.

THE PROCEDURE

The doctor may apply a numbing agent or ice to your skin, both before and after the injection. The injection of the filler material is done through a microneedle. Although several injections will be needed, depending on the size of the wrinkle or scar to be filled, discomfort should be minimal; no more than a pin prick. After the injection, the doctor may gently mold the injectable implant for the best aesthetic effect.

Lip augmentation is a different story. Because of the large number of nerves in the lips, they are very sensitive and augmentation can be quite uncomfortable, though the discomfort only lasts one or two minutes. For more details, see page 94.

HOW LONG IT TAKES

Depending on the size of the area to be treated, the procedure will take only fifteen minutes to half an hour for most injectable implants. One of the best things about injectables is that the results are literally immediate: you can see how you look right away. If you feel you need more filler, it can be done in that same session.

HOW OFTEN IT NEEDS TO BE DONE

Collagen implants, including Dermalogen, usually need to be replaced every three to six weeks, or occasionally less frequently. In contrast, most of the synthetic injectables are longer-lasting. For example, the ones that contain cross-linked hyaluronic acid, such as Reviderm and Perlane, usually last for six to eighteen months. However, it is best to avoid over-injecting, which is accomplished by giving the injections over two or three sessions, with the optimum result seen after the final session. After the series is completed, touchups, if needed, should only be required one or two times a year.

WHAT TO DO AFTER

Immediately after the procedure, the doctor may have you apply pressure to the area of injection, to stop any small amount of bleeding. Your doctor may also apply ice to minimize swelling. You should be ready to go back to work shortly after your injection. Bruising does occur in some patients and is usually minimal. It is more likely to occur if you have taken aspirin or vitamin E within the past few days. Any bruising or discoloration will disappear in a few days, and can be covered up with makeup, such as Dermablend.

Because injectable implants are liquids, they can be molded for up to two days after the injection. After that, they become fixed in position. It is common to have slight swelling in the area for a day or two, which will subside. It is also common to be able to feel a small nodule in the injection area with your fingertips for a few days (it is usually not visible). If it concerns you, you can reduce it with gentle to moderate finger pressure. If it doesn't reduce within two days, it will probably resolve within a month or two.

Your doctor will caution you not to unnecessarily rub the treated area for two days, and to limit strenuous exercise that involves motion of the affected area. Also, sleep on your back for the first few nights after the injection to make sure the pressure of the bed or pillow doesn't affect your new implant. If you are unable to avoid lying on your face, don't worry, as the effect will usually be minimal.

POSSIBLE SIDE EFFECTS AND CAUTIONS

With all injectables, there is always a risk of allergic reaction, though that is rare with everything but collagen. You may experience slight bruising or redness at the site of the implant, or even minor swelling. These side effects should not last more than a day or two. In rare cases, you may suffer from prolonged redness and/or itching, and even a hardening of the tissue at the injection site. If this should happen, inform your doctor.

Although also rare, several of the implant materials, especially silicone or those containing silicone, can migrate to an unwanted area, where they may form unsightly lumps. This is much less of a problem with the temporary fillers. Finally, be aware that in rare cases, the permanent injectables can cause a granuloma (a reaction to the foreign body material) to form; these are usually only a minimal problem and can be treated by local injection of a steroid. If they fail to clear up, which happens very rarely, local surgical excision is required. In extremely rare cases, the granuloma can progress and require more extensive reconstructive surgery.

Be sure to discuss all possible side effects with your doctor before beginning treatment, and make certain that you are informed of any symptoms that may indicate a possible problem.

HOW LONG UNTIL RESULTS ARE APPARENT

The effects of an injectable implant are immediate. What you see is what you get. The exception is that some of the injectables, especially collagen, may cause visible swelling when first injected. Because it's best to under-treat rather than over-treat, you may need to return for another "layer" of implants about four weeks after the first. There will be a charge for the second set of injections.

COST RANGE

Costs for injectable fillers are extremely varied, depending on the part of country where you live, where you have the procedure done, and especially the type of filler that you use. In general, you can expect a per-injection cost of between $150 (for collagen) to ten or more times that amount for some of the newer inert fillers. The fillers based on hyaluronic acid, such as Reviderm, can cost between $250 and $1,500 per injection. Dermalogen generally costs around $1,200 per area to fill, while the typical cost for a single Gore-Tex implant is around $2,000. Most costly of all is autologous fat, because it requires liposuction in addition to the injection. Prices may range from $2,400 to $6,000 or more, depending on how much fat is extracted and used. You can get a good idea of the current range of costs for the different implant materials by checking the Web (see Appendix B).

Although the costs vary widely, much more important is choosing the type of implant that your doctor feels is most appropriate for you and your particular needs. Be sure to discuss these matters as well as costs, before scheduling a treatment.

injectable implants

type of implant	how long it lasts	advantages	disadvantages
recommended			
Reviderm (hyaluronic acid + dextran microbeads)	6–18 months	Temporary but long-lasting; minimal chance of allergy	No FDA approval
Rofilan (hyaluronic acid)	6–9 months	Temporary but long-lasting; minimal chance of allergy	No FDA approval
Perlane (hyaluronic acid)	6–9 months	Temporary but long-lasting; minimal chance of allergy	No FDA approval
Restylane (Hyaluronic acid)	6–9 months	Temporary but long-lasting; minimal chance of allergy	No FDA approval
Evolution (polyvinyl microspheres in hyaluronic acid gel)	Permanent	Minimal chance of allergy	Slight possibility of granuloma. No FDA approval
New-Fill (polylactic acid)	3–18 months	Very low reaction rate	None
use with care			
Artecoll	Permanent	None	Slight possibility of granuloma. Allergic reaction to collagen very rare. No FDA approval.
Gore-Tex	Permanent and reversible	Feels soft and can be removed surgically	Can feel and look stiff under the skin.
Dermalogen (processed human tissue)	6 months to 2 years or more	Very low chance of allergy	Not removable
generally not recommended			
Silicone	Permenant	Inexpensive; soft, natural feel	Can migrate or leave lumps; remote chance of granuloma
Collagen*	3–4 months	Inexpensive; natural feel	Needs pretest for allergy
Autologous Fat	2–6 months	Your own fat	Rarely hardens; very expensive.

*Contraindications: use with care if you have a history of collagen vascular disease such as lupus, or a history of allergy to collagen.

Acupuncture Facelifts

Chinese medicine is almost mainstream these days, with *Qi* treatments offered at many clinics and Chinese herbs becoming a mainstay in health stores. The ancient Chinese system of acupuncture has become a tool in many mainstream doctors' offices, and is now accepted as an important pain reliever for some medical and dental procedures as well as in helping patients to recover from some surgeries and other procedures.

The latest twenty-first century use for this ancient practice is in the field of rejuvenation, with acupuncture facelifts joining the long list of available rejuvenation treatments. Practitioners claim that these treatments can help your body reabsorb signs of aging, like wrinkles and splotches, by balancing your body's energy channels. The acupuncture specialist may also prescribe dietary changes and herbal supplements.

According to Andy Wong, M.D., a physician who offers rejuvenating treatments in Tokyo, acupuncture improves the Qi, or life force, and balances the *Yin* and *Yang*, forces believed to be important in Chinese medicine. These energy flows can be regulated via various channels called meridians, which run through the whole body.

Yin and Yang are considered essential in maintaining optimal functioning of our organs, including the skin. Acupuncture can be used to improve the balance and flow of Qi through the meridians that travel through the face. Acne, for instance, is considered to be the result of Qi stagnation. Yellowish, dull skin tone with poor skin texture are caused by the poor flow of blood through the face. Stimulation of acupuncture points results in improvement of both Qi and blood. Suitable acupuncture points can be selectively stimulated to improve the skin tone and texture, and to produce general tightening and brightening of the face.

Although no controlled studies have been done, many recipients of this therapy swear by it. Be aware, though, that it isn't cheap. A full range of acupuncture rejuvenation treatments can run from $2,000 to $3,000 or more in major cities.

New and Emerging Treatments

In addition to the treatments we discuss in this chapter, research is constantly finding new ways to turn back the aging clock. Here are the new anti-aging weapons being developed:

- **Human Skin Growth Factor.** Under the name Repifermin, or Keratinocyte Growth Factor 2 (KGF-2), this natural healing compound is being marketed not only for medical purposes but also to stimulate growth of tissues such as collagen that become depleted and sluggish with age.
- **Isolagen.** This space-age product, currently undergoing tests but not yet widely available or approved by the FDA, is an injectable substance cultured from your own cells that reportedly stimulates growth of natural collagen exactly where it is needed. Because it is made from your own tissues, it should be allergy- and side effect-free, and is expected (but not proved) to be very long-lasting.

The way it works is that your doctor takes a small biopsy from the back of your ear and sends it to Isolagen's laboratory, where the cells are cultured and then processed into a solution of collagen-growing cells. Because it is still so new, the long-term effects are unknown. It is also one of the more expensive injectable options, costing $1,500 or more per injection.

Isolagen plans in the future to offer cryogenic storage of tissue taken while you are young to be used in later years to rebuild the deeper layers of your skin when they are needed. For further information, visit Isolagen's web site, listed in Appendix B.

chapter six
rejuvenating
light treatments

I t is ironic that sunlight is the cause of so many signs of aging, yet other forms of light are among the most effective treatments for nearly all these same symptoms. The field of light therapy, which includes lasers and Intense Pulsed Light (IPL), is among the most exciting and dynamic in the treatment of aging skin.

laser treatments

Unlike the sun, which provides "white" light—light that includes all wavelengths (colors)—a laser creates a beam of high-intensity light of one precise wavelength. Lasers have been used in industry for over forty years and are becoming increasingly important in medical applications because they can be targeted exclusively on specific areas or tissues, depending on the wavelength of the light. Thus, one type of laser can be targeted exclusively to obliterate a brown age spot, while another inactivates hair follicles beneath the skin's surface, thereby reducing the amount of hair in areas that should be bare.

Each type of medical laser is named for the type of material that creates its specific wavelength. For example, a CO_2 laser uses carbon dioxide gas, while a YAG-erbium laser uses a crystal made from yttrium, aluminum, garnet, and erbium. In plastic surgery, CO_2 and YAG-erbium lasers have long been used for mild to deep peels. They resurface the skin by vaporizing the top layers; when new skin grows, it is smoother and less blemished.

The CO_2 laser is primarily used for deep peels and the YAG-erbium laser is used for intermediate depth peels. Because they penetrate into the deeper layers of the skin, these peels can stimulate new collagen formation. However, the treatments are painful and expensive, and while the results can sometimes be very gratifying, they can occasionally cause permanent damage to your skin. Treatment with the YAG-erbium laser can lead to weeks if not months of downtime; with the CO_2 laser, months to even more than a year of downtime are expected. These lasers leave your face raw and bloody, which is why the recovery is prolonged; moreover, during the recovery period, the risk of infection is high.

The gentler treatments, however, often give excellent results, while removing most of the risk and eliminating the downtime. They are virtually painless and don't harm the surface of the skin. The downside is that the procedures usually require multiple treatments and often take a few weeks to a few months to achieve optimal results. Note that the laser treatments discussed in this chapter are considered cosmetic and are therefore not covered by insurance.

Among the currently available lasers that we recommend:

COOLTOUCH

Treatment with a CoolTouch laser is very different from a laser peel; it actually provides a way to restructure the skin from the inside out. CoolTouch and the newer CoolTouch II lasers make use of a Neodymium: YAG-erbium laser combined with a cooling spray that protects the outer layers of skin while the laser heats the dermis, about one-half millimeter below the surface of the skin. The laser targets the deeper skin layers, where it induces the growth of new collagen and elastin. CoolTouch II is a much less aggressive option than earlier laser treatments for improving generalized aging signs anywhere on the face (and other parts of the body).

Louisa, a physician of fifty-two, began using CoolTouch nearly five years ago. A strikingly beautiful woman with model-like looks, Louisa depends on her appearance to reassure patients as well as to project a youthful image for the medical conferences she often addresses. "When I was in my mid-forties, I started noticing changes in my neck and jowls," she said. "Instead of being a smooth curve, my jaw started to turn into a rectangle."

Louisa knew the risks associated with plastic surgery and decided to have CoolTouch treatments instead. The improvements were almost immediately noticeable. As CoolTouch stimulated new collagen, the skin was tightened and plumped up, firming the jaw line.

How it works. Instead of burning off surface imperfections, the CoolTouch laser actually rejuvenates the deeper layers of your skin. A protective cooling spray is applied very briefly to your skin's surface, cooling it. An instant later the laser beam fires and passes through your outer skin (epidermis), which, because it has been pre-cooled, is not harmed. The upper part of your dermis, which has not been cooled, is heated enough to cause a mild injury that stimulates the cells that produce natural collagen and elastin (fibroblasts). These cells will continue to produce new collagen and elastin for months after your treatments, leading to firmer, more elastic, and smoother skin that will increasingly appear more youthful.

In addition to stimulating collagen formation, the CoolTouch noticeably reduces wrinkles and fine lines, softens crow's feet around the eyes, and reduces the prominence of stretch marks and acne scars. It can even diminish active acne in many cases. Unlike some other treatments, it doesn't cause uneven skin pigmentation and will cause your skin to become noticeably softer to the touch. When combined with microdermabrasion to remove surface spots and imperfections, the CoolTouch II laser can truly seem a fountain of youth, restoring the soft, unblemished, and firm complexion of youth.

We recommend the CoolTouch II laser over the CoolTouch because the CoolTouch II covers a four-times-larger treatment area and is even more powerful and faster-acting than the original CoolTouch. Although our patients report that it produces noticeably more discomfort, they also prefer it for its long-lasting and much quicker results. "The good thing is that as soon as the pulse stops, so does the discomfort," said one of our patients. "I would definitely do it again, as many times as it takes."

What to do before. You will meet with your doctor a week or two before the treatment to discuss the procedure and your expectations. At that time you should ask any questions you have about the procedure or the equipment, and your physician will tell you what improvement you can realistically expect. He will also caution you to avoid sunburn and to refrain from using any abrasive products on your face before your appointment. You should also discontinue use of Renova or any other Retin-A product for several days before the treatment. This precaution is because an active sunburn or current Renova treatment causes inflammation of the skin; it is best to let this inflammation reduce over a few days before the CoolTouch laser treatment.

The procedure. A half-hour to an hour before your treatment, the doctor will apply a numbing cream to the site of the laser treatment. When the numbing agent has taken effect, it will be washed off and your face dried, then you will be seated in a comfortable chair that resembles a dentist's chair. You and everyone else in the treatment room, including the doctor, will be given protective goggles to shield your eyes from the bright flash of the laser.

Before beginning, your doctor will use the photometer attached to the laser to measure your skin temperature, then fire a single pulse from the laser, which first sprays the cooling agent, then applies a quick laser pulse. You will hear a short, sharp buzzing sound when the laser pulses, and will feel a warm or slight burning sensation in the area of treatment, sometimes described as feeling like a rubber band snap against your skin.

Immediately after applying the pulse, a meter on the CoolTouch laser will indicate the maximum temperature of your skin surface, and whether or not it is in the treatment range; the doctor might have to do several test pulses to achieve the proper treatment range. The treatment will then continue in a series of closely spaced pulses every 0.8 seconds, each one preceded by the cooling spray, until the entire area has been treated. This single treatment works best for deeper wrinkles and scars.

For more superficial, finer lines and wrinkles, the CoolTouch II may be used to make a second pass; first heating, then instantly cooling the epidermis.

After your treatment, you may be given a cooling icepack to apply on the treated areas for ten or fifteen minutes, and may be given a prescription for a soothing lotion. The area treated may feel warm and appear pink, usually for less than two hours. You will also be urged to wear at least 15 SPF sunscreen whenever you expose your face to the sun. This is a good idea for everyone anyway.

How long it takes. An average CoolTouch treatment takes 15 to 30 minutes, depending on how much of your face (or other part of your body) is treated. If you only want a quick touch-up—say, of the wrinkles around your eyes—

the treatment can take as little as ten minutes. It is so quick and easy you can actually have it done on your lunch hour. If you decide to have topical anesthesia, it is most effective if it is left on for at least 30 minutes. To save time, the doctor may prescribe this for you to apply at home.

How often it needs to be done. An initial series of three or four treatments, performed three to six weeks apart, with only occasional maintenance treatments thereafter will give optimum results. Although the natural collagen produced by CoolTouch II will last for years, one or two touch-up treatments yearly will help maintain the results.

Possible side effects and cautions. The momentary discomfort produced by the laser pulse disappears as soon as the pulse ends. After your treatment, you can expect to see a slight to moderate reddening in the area that was treated. This should fade within an hour or so, and you can apply makeup immediately if you wish.

How long until results are apparent. Most patients report an improvement in both their skin tone and texture within a couple of months following the first treatment. These beneficial results will continue, growing even greater, for several more months. Be aware that CoolTouch II will not affect superficial blemishes and age spots. To quickly improve the appearance and texture of your complexion, Renova, Kinerase, or microdermabrasion can be used in conjunction with CoolTouch.

Cost range. Depending on where you have the procedure done and the extent of the area you have treated, the cost for a single CoolTouch or CoolTouch II treatment should range between $250 and $1000 or more. Many doctors offer a reduced rate for a series of treatments.

NLITE LASER COLLAGEN REPLENISHMENT

Nlite, a yellow pulse-dye laser that is designed specifically to stimulate the formation of new collagen, is one of a number of new rejuvenating laser devices. Like the CoolTouch, the Nlite stimulates the collagen-producing cells by causing a mild thermal injury beneath the wrinkles in the top layers of skin. The CoolTouch laser wavelength is absorbed by water, the Nlite by small blood vessels; the net result in both is a mild thermal injury that stimulates collagen formation. Nlite was approved by the FDA in 2000 for treatment of periocular (around the eye) wrinkles, but because it produces such good results, many doctors are using it for full-face treatments.

Since it is so gentle, Nlite treatments will work for most people, although you should discuss the possibilities thoroughly with your doctor if you have dark skin that tends to form hyperpigmentation or keloids. Nlite is *not* recommended for those with active herpes, warts, acne, rosacea, or autoimmune disorders. Based on the experience of doctors who pioneered the Nlite in Britain, it works best for those who are under 55, although older patients will also see good results.

How it works. The energy of the yellow laser Nlite passes harmlessly through the upper layers of your skin, producing no burning or pain. The Nlite wavelength is absorbed by small blood vessels, which, in turn, heat the surrounding tissue and, much like CoolTouch, the heat created stimulates the growth of new collagen and elastin in the deeper layers of the skin, plumping the skin up and reducing the depth and appearance of surface wrinkles.

What to do before. Since Nlite is relatively new, it is essential to make sure that your doctor is experienced in its use. Improperly applied Nlite (turned too high or applied too long) can result in bruising and dark marks on the skin. At present, Nlite is not available in all areas of the country. The Nlite machine is not available for purchase; instead, doctors rent it for a day or two at a time.

To avoid bruising, your doctor will probably advise you not to take aspirin, ibuprofen, Alleve, or vitamin E for a week prior to your treatment.

Don't use facial scrubs or alcohol-based cleansers prior to your treatment. Also, it's best to refrain from vigorous physical activity at least two hours before receiving Nlite treatments. Be sure to remove all traces of makeup and other cosmetics, such as sunscreens, from your face at least thirty minutes prior to the procedure.

The procedure. You will be seated in a reclining medical chair and given protective goggles before the procedure begins (along with everyone else in the treatment room). The doctor will then apply the Nlite laser to your face, repeatedly targeting small sectors in the wrinkled areas that you wish to rejuvenate. One great advantage to Nlite treatments is that they are virtually painless, though some people experience a transient sensation of warmth.

How long it takes. Depending on the number and severity of your wrinkles, a full-face treatment should take between twenty minutes and an hour. For best results, it's recommended that you receive a second treatment approximately two weeks after the first.

How often it needs to be done. Most doctors recommend two treatments (spaced two weeks apart). Once new collagen has formed, it will remain for up to several years. However, be aware that you must still protect your skin (avoid the sun, wear sunscreen) and that eventually you will need further treatments.

What to do after. Because the procedure is painless and causes no side effects, there is no recovery time and you are free to put on sunscreen and makeup and go about your daily life. For three to four days after your treatment, you may be asked not to perform any strenuous exercise. No other follow-up treatment is necessary, however.

Possible side effects and cautions. There are virtually no immediate side effects from treatment with Nlite: no redness, burning, or other irritation. Very rarely, some patients have reported slight, transient swelling, which can be relieved with ice. Unlike some procedures, Nlite does not increase your sun sensitivity, though you should still wear a strong SPF sunscreen after the procedure and any time you go out into the sun.

How long until results are apparent. Most patients begin to see results within a month or so of their first treatment, as the new collagen is formed and its effects become visible. Optimum results should be achieved within three to four months.

Cost range. As with most relatively new cosmetic procedures, costs for Nlite treatment can vary, depending on how much treatment you require and the part of the country where you have the procedure done. Although Nlite is not as widely available as some other laser treatment options, you can find practitioners in most major metro areas. Costs are usually based on a full-face treatment, for which you may be charged anywhere from $800 to more than $1,200 for a treatment (some doctors will offer a package deal for two treatments, expect to pay at least $2,000). Some doctors charge by the treatment area, with $400 to 800 for the eyes as a representative price range.

comparing lasers

Our experience suggests that the CoolTouch II is more effective than the Nlite, similar lasers such as the SmoothBeam, manufactured by Candela, any of the other competing non-ablative lasers, or IPL for the stimulation of collagen and reducing wrinkles. But the laser field is in a continual state of development and improvement. Incidentally, the CoolTouch laser and the Nlite laser are now made by the same company, ICN, Inc.

SPECIALIZED LASERS

A growing number of specialized lasers are available for cosmetic treatments. For the most part, each laser is best suited to a particular procedure, such as fading red marks or zapping hair follicles. Some lasers can be adjusted to be used for more than one purpose. Using the wrong laser or using it incorrectly can result in skin damage that can be severe and even disfiguring.

When using a laser for cosmetic purposes, an experienced practitioner must find the ideal combination of laser wavelength, energy intensity, type and degree of cooling, and exposure time. For example, when lasers are applied too slowly to an area, adjacent tissue can be damaged, resulting in scarring. When the laser's energy is applied too fast, the small blood vessels in the area can literally explode, causing severe bruising. Many laser systems offer computer-assisted adjustments for each patient. Make certain that the laser your doctor proposes to use is approved for the area you wish treated, and be certain that he or she is experienced in the use of that particular laser. Don't be afraid to ask your doctor for all details on the laser he is planning to use for your treatment. For more information on finding a qualified doctor for laser treatments, see chapter 9.

AURA AND SIMILAR LASERS

This type of KTP (potassium-titanyl-phosphate) laser (Aura is manufactured by Laserscope) produces green light (532 nm). It is used to erase red and brown spots, such as birthmarks, moles, skin tags, and age spots anywhere on the body. It is very effective at removing spider veins and rosacea on the face (see chapter 8 for details). The Aura laser is also used for spider and varicose veins up to 4 mm in diameter on the legs, especially those that are red in color, although it is not the first choice for treatment (because it can cause bruising). A caveat: the Aura and similar lasers are more likely to cause complications, including superficial burning, darkening, or lightening of the skin, if you have darker or suntanned skin.

LYRA LASER

Also manufactured by Laserscope, this laser is used widely for hair removal (for more details see chapter 15). The Lyra laser produces near-infrared "light" that is invisible. The light passes through a transparent tip that is chilled to near zero degrees Celsius, protecting the skin and reducing discomfort. When it reaches the target area, the laser energy heats and destroys the targeted tissue. If the tissue is a hair follicle, the hair will cease to grow or grow finer and lighter; if the target is a spider vein or small varicose vein, it is injured and then eventually absorbed by the body.

Because of its long wavelength and pulsed light, the Lyra is said to be extremely safe and has been approved by the FDA for use with all skin types and colors, even naturally dark or suntanned skin, without affecting pigmentation. It is considered one of the best choices for all skin colors, both for hair removal and the treatment of spider veins on the legs. It has recently been approved by the FDA for treatment of fine wrinkles on the face.

> **Note:** The following description of the procedure for the Aura laser and the before and after suggestions hold true for most laser treatments. The only difference, apart from the fact that different lasers target different tissues, is that some laser treatments may be slightly more uncomfortable than others.

What to do before. Your doctor may have you hold ice on the treatment area for a few minutes before the procedure to cool the skin and numb any slight discomfort.

The procedure. For facial treatments, you will be seated in a comfortable reclining medical chair. As with any laser procedure, you will be given goggles to protect your eyes from the bright flash caused when the laser pulses. It is also a good idea to keep your eyes closed during the procedure. The doctor will position the laser and pulse it as many times as necessary to obliterate the targeted blemish, moving the laser beam between pulses to cover the targeted areas.

The Aura is so fast that many patients report the treatment is completely painless, while others describe a momentary sensation akin to a hot pinprick.

	light rejuvenation devices			
name	**trade name/ manufacturer**	**type**	**use**	**similar lasers**
Aura	Laserscope	KTP laser with parallel cooling	Red and brown spots; broken veins; used primarily on light-colored skin from the neck up.	Versapulse (Coherent; discontinued)
CoolTouch II	ICN	Low-energy infrared laser	Stimulates collagen growth, restores skin texture	Older model CoolTouch
GentleLASE	Candela	Alexandrite laser	Red spots, tattoos, hair removal	Apogee
Nlite	ICN Medical Alliance	Pulsed-dye laser	Stimulates the formation of collagen	SmoothBeam (Candela)
Lyra	Laserscope	i-Nd: YAG laser with parallel cooling	Hair removal in all skin colors; spider veins and small varicose veins on the legs and elsewhere; skin rejuvenation on the face.	Varia (ICN)
Intense Pulsed LIght (IPL)	Vasculite (Photoderm)	Intense broad-spectrum light	Skin discoloration, red blemishes, Rosacea; restores skin texture, hair removal	Fotofacial (Infini), Estelux (Palomar), Multilight (Photoderm)

How long it takes. Most Aura procedures can be completed in your doctor's office in no more than fifteen or thirty minutes.

What to do after. Because the Aura laser is used on light skin types, it's important to avoid direct sunlight as much as possible for 36 hours and to wear sunscreen. If the treatment is for spider or varicose veins on your legs (using Aura or Lyra lasers), avoid both alcohol and aspirin for a few days, as alcohol can cause the blood vessels to dilate and aspirin causes delayed clotting of the blood—either of these will increase the chance of bruising and recurrence of the treated vessels.

Possible side effects and cautions. Complications are all but nonexistent with Aura therapy. Very rarely, you may notice a lightening of pigment around the treated area, which should return to normal within a few months.

How long until results are apparent. For small blemishes, such as moles, the results are apparent immediately after the procedure, though there may be a small red spot at the site of the treatment for up to several weeks. For larger areas, such as large birthmarks or spider or varicose veins on the leg, repeat treatments may be necessary.

Costs. The cost of an Aura treatment depends on the area being treated and how many treatments are necessary. Costs for facial treatment, such as the cheeks and nose, average $300 to $500 (somewhat more in major urban areas). Be sure to discuss costs as well as payment options with your doctor.

PHOTOREJUVENATION: INTENSE PULSED LIGHT

Used extensively in Asia and Europe, photorejuvenation, or Intense Pulsed Light therapy (IPL), is a new nonsurgical treatment that is said by its proponents to work wonders on aging skin. Rather than using a laser, which applies an intense beam of a specific light frequency to the targeted part of the skin, IPL uses intense pulses of broad-spectrum light—white light that contains many different wavelengths—to deliver light energy, which is immediately converted to heat, to the skin or beneath the skin, depending on the desired outcome of the treatment. The treatment is often adjustable by use of various filters, making this procedure effective for a wide range of skin types.

How it works. Like CoolTouch laser treatments, IPL works by rapid heating of the targeted tissue, and it can stimulate formation of new collagen beneath the skin. However, because it contains more than one wavelength of light, it can affect several aging signs at the same time. Thus, at the same treatment session, IPL can remove redness, broken capillaries, and fine lines; shrink large pores; and diminish acne scars. It can be used to improve an aging appearance on the entire face, as well as the neck, chest, and backs of the hands. IPL can also remove unwanted hair. It is said to be effective also in removing tattoos and treating rosacea.

> **Note:** IPL does not improve frown lines, especially on the fore-head and between the eyebrows; baggy or sagging skin; puffi-ness around the eyes; drooping eyelids; bumpy moles (though it will remove their pigment); skin cancers (though it can treat pre-cancerous lesions); seborrheic keratoses; or deep acne scars (though it will soften shallow scars).

What to do before. Two or more weeks before the procedure, you will meet with your doctor for a pre-consultation during which your doctor will ascertain the general state of your health and discuss your expectations from the treatment. She will also take a medical history. IPL is not considered suitable for patients with connective tissue diseases such as lupus and some forms of arthritis. You should not have IPL if you are pregnant, have a recent suntan or sunburn, or are planning non-routine sun exposure (or a tanning booth treat-ment) in the weeks after the treatment. Insulin-dependent diabetics are also ineligible for this treatment because of the remote possibility of blistering or other damage, since diabetics experience difficulty in healing.

To determine if you are a good candidate for IPL, you will undergo a patch test—applying the IPL to a small patch of your skin—to make sure that you don't suffer any adverse reactions, such as blistering, redness, irritation, or hyperpigmentation. You will have to sign an informed consent form and pay for this preliminary test. Assuming you have no adverse reactions to this test, you can schedule your appointment for the actual treatment. You will be instructed not to take any medications that might thin your blood (and increase the likelihood of bleeding), such as aspirin and vitamin E, and told to stay out of the sun until after the procedure.

On the day of the procedure, do not shave or use any cosmetics. If you have active herpes or a skin infection present on the day of treatment, the treatment will be postponed until the condition clears up.

The procedure. IPL can sting when it's being applied. A numbing cream can be applied 30 to 60 minutes beforehand to reduce discomfort. When your treatment is ready to begin, you will be seated in a medical chair and a sooth-ing gel will be applied to the treatment area. You will be given protective gog-gles, and then a glass prism in the shape of a pyramid will be placed against the area to be treated first. The bright pulsed light is flashed onto your skin through the prism, which is moved as many times as necessary to cover the entire affected area.

How long it takes. A whole-face treatment usually takes about thirty minutes, and a series of four to six treatments, spaced four to six weeks apart, is usually recommended.

How often it needs to be done. The results are long-lasting, but you will need occasional touchup treatments, from every several months to every year or two.

What to do after. Sometimes ice is applied to the treatment area afterward. You will be instructed to stay out of the sun and wear a sunscreen of at least 30 SPF.

Possible side effects and cautions. Although your face may appear quite pink and even somewhat puffy after IPL treatment, you can go back to your daily routine immediately. Be sure to notify your doctor if the redness doesn't disappear within a very few days.

Why I Prefer IPL
by Dr. Joseph Georghy,
Director of North Shore Cosmetic, Sydney, Australia

In Australia, a large percentage of the population has fair skin, easily damaged by the sun. Intense Pulsed Light (IPL) can easily, quickly, and effectively treat most of these common problems, including redness and broken capillaries, fine wrinkles, poor skin tone, age spots, large pores, unwanted facial hair, birth marks, acne and acne scarring, rosacea, and rough, coarse-looking skin.

IPL is particularly good at eliminating unwanted reddening of the skin, no matter what its cause. In some cases the skin has an overall reddish tinge with no blood vessels visible, but IPL emissions can find even the tiniest blood vessels and eliminate them.

No other procedure can accomplish so much with such low risk and no downtime. My patients assure me the discomfort is minimal to non-existent, and they appreciate that they can have it done literally as a lunchtime procedure. The patient satisfaction rate is more than 90 percent.

Very rarely, patients experience blistering or even minor bleeding from IPL treatments. Some dark-skinned patients can experience pigment changes, which usually disappear within a few weeks to months.

How long until results are apparent. It will take a while for the full benefits of each IPL treatment to develop, from a few weeks to a few months.

Cost range. Costs for IPL are generally more than microdermabrasion but less than laser treatment. They vary depending on where you have the treatment done and how many pulses you need. A patch test usually costs between $25 and $75. Pulses usually cost around $10 each, with a usual minimum of $100. Count on spending at least $100 per treatment.

IPL machines. A number of companies make IPL machines; among the best known are Vasculite, Fotofacial, Estelux, and Multilight.

The Vasculite Plus, made by PhotoDerm, is said to be the most advanced system. Operated by a sophisticated computer, the Vasculite combines a number of laser capabilities to treat a number of different skin problems (including excess hair) on a wide variety of skin types.

ThermaCool TC

New on the market is the ThermaCool TC system, an FDA-approved device manufactured by ThermAge. The innovation in this device is the use of continually monitored contact cooling through a membrane in the treatment tip that is placed in contact with the skin. Radiofrequency (RF) is also delivered through the treatment tip, and sensors measure the pressure of the tip on the skin and the skin temperature. The device can control the depth of tissue heating and thereby cause a controlled thermal injury. The mechanism of action is tissue tightening by heating up the molecular bonds in collagen with consequent contraction of the collagen. Studies have shown benefit in the non-invasive treatment of periorbital rhytids and wrinkles, as well as in ameloriating active acne. Preliminary results also suggest that tightening of the skin occurs, which might help with a non-invasive minifacelift, such as reducing sagging jowls. This is also a lunchtime treatment with no downtime. However, there is some discomfort during the treatment and oral medication is often used to reduce pain and for sedation.

---

chapter seven

putting it all together: combination treatments

For people with profound aging changes or high-profile careers, the most satisfactory results are obtained by combining various treatments and products. In deciding on an individualized approach for a person, we look on the available treatments almost as if they were different colors in an artist's palette, then combine them to achieve a "picture-perfect" result.

Some of the treatments we offer, for example, can minimize fine lines and wrinkles, while others are better suited for plumping out deep furrows. Some treatments are extremely good at removing surface spots and blemishes, yet do nothing for sags and bags. We find that when we use these treatments in conjunction with each other, each improvement actually enhances the other.

using botox to enhance other procedures

One of the most common and effective combinations is the use of Botox with a number of other treatments. We and other physicians increasingly find that Botox improves the outcome of other procedures, especially those involving areas where muscle movement is an important factor. For example, by relaxing muscles and helping the face to become more in balance, without greater muscle stress on one side than the other, Botox generally makes it easier to offer more accurate, balanced, and esthetically pleasing treatments.

INJECTABLE IMPLANTS

Another important use for Botox is in conjunction with injectable implants. Not only can the implants sometimes enhance Botox therapy, use of Botox can make the implants more effective. Useful as they are, the implants are mainly liquid, and subject to slight movement for hours to a few days after they are injected. This is good, in that they can then be gently molded into the best position and shape. But it's also a problem, because if you sleep with pressure on the implant before it has fixed in place, it might move or mold in an unwanted way. Muscle action can also displace the implant. To avoid the former problem, sleep on your back for two days. To avoid the latter, ask your doctor to combine the implants with Botox, which weakens the muscles and reduces any movement of the implant away from the crevice or line it was intended to fill.

We particularly like to use Botox as an adjunctive treatment with injectable implants for nasolabial folds, marionette lines, and other deep wrinkles. By weakening the muscle that causes the line or crease, Botox can help the injectable implant to stay precisely where it was implanted.

DEEP PEELS

Although we do not advocate deep peels or laser resurfacing, those who have resurfacing of the upper part of the face will have a much better result if they are pre-treated with Botox. Using Botox to relax the muscles responsible for crow's feet, frown lines, and "bunny" lines (creases on the sides and top of the nose that happen with expression) can prevent the wrinkling from quickly returning to the newly resurfaced skin.

In addition to pretreatment, a recent study demonstrated that using Botox

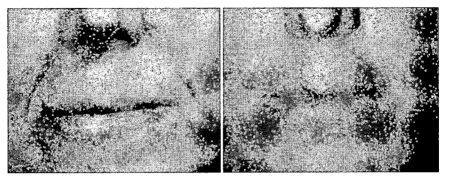

Pretreatment (Left)
After injectable implant and CoolTouch laser (Right)

after resurfacing can not only improve the appearance of the new skin, it also prevents or delays recurrence of the unwanted wrinkles and furrows.

EYELID SURGERY

Another area in which Botox is increasingly used is eyelid surgery, or ble-pharoplasty. Typically, this operation involves cutting away excess skin and fat from the upper or lower eyelids or both. In some cases, the muscles are tight-ened as well. By pre-treating the crow's feet extending from the corners of the eyelids, resulting in more relaxed eye muscles, your doctor can work more accu-rately, which improves the result after surgery. Pretreatment with Botox also makes any scars less visible.

NECK SURGERY

Dr. Alan Matarasso, a New York plastic surgeon who pioneered some cosmetic uses of Botox, likes to use Botox as an adjunct to neck surgery. "It's good for getting the things surgery didn't correct," he reports.

In our own practice, we find Botox extremely useful both as a stand-alone treatment and in conjunction with other procedures. In addition to those men-tioned already, we also use Botox in conjunction with CoolTouch laser treat-ments (see chapter 6). CoolTouch minimizes deep and superficial wrinkles, but does nothing for the underlying problem of hyperactive muscles, which is, so to speak, the specialty of Botox.

DEEP LINES AND SCARS

Injectable implants are also used in conjunction with deep peels for sunken facial scars, such as those caused by acne. After the implant is injected, "laser skin resurfacing is used following the procedure to soften any remaining lines."

Although we avoid invasive procedures such as resurfacing, we use similar combinations, such as implants with Botox or CoolTouch for wrinkles and sags; we often add microdermabrasion or superficial peels to improve the skin's texture and appearance. Remember that the changes caused by the sun, environmental damage, and aging are complex, and minimizing or eliminating them is often complex also. In addition to all the treatments we've described so far, new rejuvenating products and tools are constantly being developed.

The chart on the next page summarizes the uses of some of the treatments and products we recommend, indicating their most effective use.

When Plastic Surgery May Be Necessary

We truly believe that with the great new treatments we describe in this book, most old-fashioned plastic surgery procedures are all but obsolete. In most cases, using rejuvenating treatments can prevent the need for plastic surgery or at worst postpone it. It can also, as this chapter demonstrates, improve the results of most plastic surgery.

However, there are some situations that still require plastic surgery for the best aesthetic effect. Though many of the treatments described in this book can help these conditions, only surgery can eliminate them. The most common of these conditions are:

- **Heavy jowls** That "jowly" look can often be minimized with Botox, injectable implants, and the ThermaCool machine. However, due in some cases to heredity, some people develop very obvious and obtrusive jowls that can best be treated through surgery.
- **Fallen neck** Botox and injectable implants can all but eliminate the ugly, scrawny "turkey neck" that so many of us experience in middle age. However, fallen neck, in which large fatty deposits form in the center of the neck, can only be alleviated by removing the fatty deposits through liposuction. Sometimes surgery is also required to get rid of excess skin in the area.
- **Droopy eyelids and fatty bags under the eyes** Botox can work wonders for old and tired-looking eyes, but if your eyelids droop markedly (a hereditary trait), or if you develop noticeable fatty bags under your eyes, your best option is blepharoplasty, or eyelid surgery, which can completely eliminate both problems.

---

comparing cosmetic products and procedures

treatment or product	dynamic deep wrinkles	static deep wrinkles	fine lines	sagging skin	neck bands	spots, blemishes, rosacea, visible vessels
Botox	+++++	+	+++	+	+++	−
Injectable implants	++++	++++	+++	++	++	−
CoolTouch	+	+++	++++	++	++	−
Aura laser (green lasers)	−	+	+	+	−	+++++
Intense pulsed light (IPL)	+	+++	+++	++	+	++++
Microderma-brasion	−	+	++	−	−	+++
Plastic surgery	++	+++	++	++++	++++	−
Deep peel	++	+++	+++	++	−	++++
Renova	−	++	+++	+	−	++
Kinerase	−	+	++	−	−	+
Vitamin C	−	+	+	+	−	−
Copper Cream	−	+	++	+	−	+

Key: +++++ Excellent results
+++++ Good to excellent results
+++ Good results
++ Fair to good results
+ Fair results
− No effect

81

.

chapter eight

specific
solutions for
specific
problems

In previous chapters, we've addressed methods of dealing with the most common and disturbing signs of aging: wrinkles, sags, and discoloration. There are many other cosmetic problems, however, some connected with aging, and some not, that can also be solved through relatively painless, nonsurgical means. In this chapter, we'll take a look at a variety of these problems and explain how to solve them.

getting the spots out

We discussed the use of a number of treatments to get rid of wrinkles. We also mentioned the ugly spots that can proliferate on your face, arms, and hands after a certain age. Let's take a closer look at some of these spots, most of which respond as if by magic to a variety of treatments we've already recommended, including Renova, glycolic and alpha-hydroxy acids, laser and light therapy, and microdermabrasion, as well as a variety of face of over-the-counter preparations such as Triluma and Kinerase (discussed in chapter 10).

AGE SPOTS

Next to wrinkles, the proliferation of ugly brown spots is among the most common and least-liked results of aging. Caused primarily by exposure to sunlight, these flat, ugly blotches, also called liver spots and senile lentigos, are essentially concentrated areas of melanin, the skin's dark pigment. Not surprisingly, they are usually most prominent on the face, neck, chest, hands, and forearms, where there has been greatest exposure to the elements.

These ugly spots can be faded or eliminated by nearly all the procedures and products we've mentioned previously, including Renova, microdermabrasion, and laser and light treatments. A bonus of having your wrinkles wiped out by these methods is that they usually zap your brown spots too.

SEBORRHEIC KERATOSES

These repulsive splotches, also caused by age and exposure to the sun, are usually found in the same sun-exposed areas as age spots. Unlike the flat, freckle-like age spots, though, seborrheic keratoses are warty, and raised. They often look as if they have been stuck onto your skin's surface with glue. They are usually brown, but can be gray or yellow, and often have an oily appearance.

Although they can look even worse than age spots, seborrheic keratoses are completely harmless. They are essentially concentrated clumps of melanin pigment, and the tendency to develop them seems to run in families. They most commonly appear on the neck and trunk, though they can also appear elsewhere, including the face. In rare cases, seborrheic keratoses can mask serious skin cancers. If you develop these unsightly blotches, it's best to see a dermatologist, who will biopsy them if necessary, or quickly remove with them by freezing or zapping them with a laser if they are clearly benign.

RED BLEMISHES (HEMANGIOMATA)

These are blemishes caused by abnormal blood vessels close to the surface of the skin, which can give the skin a reddish tinge. Unlike the brown and yellow spots described above, red blemishes and discolorations are treated differently, depending on their position on the body, their size, and some other factors. The majority of them are usually treated with lasers and other light therapy. Specifics follow for each type of blemish.

How to Tell Harmless Blemishes from More Dangerous Changes That Need Medical Attention

The vast majority of spots and blemishes are harmless changes caused by aging or sunlight or both. However, a small number of such spots could actually be precancerous or even cancerous lesions. The only way to tell for sure is to see an experienced physician, who may perform a biopsy. This remote danger of skin cancer is one of the many reasons you should always have cosmetic treatments performed by a qualified and experienced medical professional.

The spots that are most likely to be precancerous lesions are technically called *actinic keratoses*, and are usually flat, dry, and scaly with a reddish appearance. They feel rough to the touch, and are most common in blondes and redheads, people who freckle, those with blue eyes, and those with Scandinavian or Scotch-Irish heritage. These lesions should be evaluated and, if necessary, removed by your doctor before you have any cosmetic procedures done.

Like other spots, actinic keratoses are more likely to appear the older you get, and they are most common in areas that already show changes due to aging, such as brown spots, wrinkles, and lack of elasticity.

Other changes that may indicate a precancerous or cancerous condition include any sores in a sun-exposed area (or even in areas not exposed to the sun) that do not heal, or continually bleed, and any spot that keeps growing in size. Be especially wary of moles that change color or size, or suddenly appear. Chances are, anything you notice is most likely a harmless aging change, but any time you notice a suspicious spot, play it safe and have it evaluated right away.

MOLES

In the past, moles have usually been surgically removed, but increasingly, lasers are used to do the job. The laser can precisely target the pigmented tissue of the mole, leading to complete removal with less chance of scarring or harming adjacent tissue. An important caution, however: serious skin cancers such as melanoma often begin in moles, so make certain that your doctor is experienced with skin lesions of all sorts. If he finds your mole suspicious, he will biopsy it before removing it. If you are prone to form keloids, be sure to discuss possible side effects with your doctor.

ACNE AND OTHER SCARS

Once a potentially disfiguring ailment, severe acne has left generations of men and women with ugly, lifelong scarring . . . until now. Brad, a forty-eight-year-old hairdresser in a high-profile Manhattan salon, had long been ashamed of the bumpy, disfiguring results of his adolescent "pizza face." Four treatments with CoolTouch laser, accompanied by injectable implants in the areas with greatest scarring, permanently smoothed Brad's face. "I looked in the mirror and cried," Brad reported after the first treatment. "For the first time since sixth grade, I liked what I saw."

Acne and other facial scars represent far more than mere blemishes. Because your face is your public representation, facial scars can cause low self-esteem and other psychological problems.

Until fairly recently, the best treatment for facial and acne scars was medium and deep peels (either chemical or laser). The problem with these peels is that they injure the skin and may take weeks to heal. In some cases, peels may still be the best option. But for most scars, less invasive, gentler methods give equally good results without pain and downtime.

Depending on the extent and depth of the scarring, CoolTouch II laser treatments can plump the scars out with your own new collagen. A series of four or five treatments, with an interval of a few weeks between treatments is optimal; a shorter interval is probably not as effective. A longer interval is fine, but it will take longer to achieve the best results. A visible improvement should be evident within two to three months, and this improvement will continue as new collagen continues to be formed within the deeper layers of the skin.

In some instances, the scarring is too extensive or deep to be erased by CoolTouch II treatments. For those deeper scars, injectable implants can provide

A cancer survivor's story

Elaine M. was shocked to be diagnosed with kidney cancer at age fifty. The divorced mother of two grown sons was at the pinnacle of her interior design career and her personal life. Now she faced an uncertain future along with the ravages of chemotherapy.

"I decided very early on in the process that I didn't want people to know I was sick," Elaine said. "I didn't want to look sick. I didn't want those knowing looks and that pity."

"I'd been thinking about having some cosmetic treatments done anyway, and now was as good a time as any," Elaine explained. "The great thing is that they don't interfere with the cancer treatments."

Because Elaine was already stressed financially and physically, she opted for a relatively simple program. She began with CoolTouch over most of her face and Botox injections around her eyes and forehead area. In addition, she had microdermabrasion every two to three months.

"It's a great morale booster," she reported. "Within a few weeks, all the brown spots on my forehead were gone and my skin was more even textured. Now people tell me how good my skin looks."

As for her intention not to look sick, Elaine succeeded beyond her dreams. A year after her diagnosis, and still in treatment, Elaine is extremely attractive, with short, streaked blond hair, beautiful smooth skin, and a lovely smile. She looks, in fact, like a vibrant, healthy forty-year old, more than ten years younger than her chronological age.

"A few months ago, I went into cardiac arrest during a chemo session," Elaine admitted. "I had to spend a few days in Intensive Care. The nurses, the doctors, the emergency technicians, all of them kept coming in to look at me. They kept saying, "You look fabulous! I can't believe you arrested!"

instant gratification by filling in the depressed area, although the results will not be as long-lasting, and repeat injections will usually be required to maintain an optimal appearance. A combination of the CoolTouch II laser and injectable implants gives longer-lasting results and more immediate gratification. Once the worst of the scarring has been eased by CoolTouch II and/or injectable fillers, microdermabrasion or superficial glycolic acid peels can further enhance your new smooth, unpitted complexion.

CoolTouch II is by far the best option for acne, treating the scars without causing uneven pigmentation on dark skin, as often happens with chemical and laser peels.

broken capillaries and spider veins

These unsightly blemishes, which are much more common, or at least more visible, in men and women with light-colored skin than in those who are darker, occur when tiny blood vessels enlarge and become visible through the skin. Technically known as *telangiectasia*, these red or purple blotches most often appear on the face, chest, and legs, though they may occur anywhere on the body.

Susceptibility to telangiectasia appears to be hereditary. It is thought to be brought on by exposure to sunlight or radiation, as well as by trauma, pressure, pregnancy, hormone replacement therapy, and simply aging. They are totally harmless from a medical perspective, but who wants weird little squiggly red lines or red dots (called cherry angiomas) or blotches?

Luckily, there are a number of quick and simple ways to completely eliminate these ugly arachnids from your life. Among the quickest are lasers that are specially designed to get the red out.

LASER TREATMENT FOR SPIDER VEINS

In the past, laser therapy wasn't very successful for eliminating these small but visibly prominent vessels because it harmed the outer skin and caused bruising beneath the skin where the capillary was destroyed. With new technology, those problems are significantly reduced: the outer skin is cooled while the blood within the capillary is targeted. The targeted tissue is superheated, destroying the vessel walls, which will eventually be resorbed by the body. In many cases, one treatment is enough to completely eliminate the spider veins, but multiple treatments of the same spider vein might well be required; in more difficult cases, two or at most three treatments might be required. Among the best-known lasers used to zap spider veins and other reddish lesions are the Versapulse from Coherent; the Varia from CoolTouch; and the Aura and Lyra from Laserscope. Lasers are discussed in more detail in chapter 6.

Who can have this procedure? Laser removal of spider veins on the face isn't for everyone; it works best for people with light, relatively untanned and unsunburned skin. This is because instead of passing harmlessly through the outer skin, the laser's energy can be absorbed by the outer layers of dark skin, causing damage. The Lyra laser is an exception; when used properly, it is considered safe for all types of skin.

specific solutions for specific problems

What to do before. For several weeks before your treatment, avoid anything more than minimal routine sun exposure. Wear an SPF 30 sunscreen in the areas to be treated. Don't wear make-up in the areas to be treated prior to treatment, although if you have already applied make-up it can be removed before your treatment.

The procedure. Although laser treatment for spider veins isn't totally painless, discomfort should be minimal. Many describe it as feeling like a rubber band repeatedly being snapped against your skin. Anesthesia isn't normally necessary, but your doctor may apply an anesthetic cream or occasionally give an injection of local anesthetic.

You will be seated in a medical reclining chair and given a pair of protective goggles (as will everyone in the room). The area to be treated will be covered with a special gel that facilitates the treatment. The doctor will then give you one or more pulses with the laser, depending on how large and how extensive your spider veins are. Afterward, the doctor may apply ice packs for a few minutes and/or apply a light coating of post-laser gel to soothe the area treated.

How long it takes. Treatment should last from a few minutes for a small spider vein to around 30 minutes or more for larger varicose veins, multiple spider veins, or clusters of veins.

How often it needs to be done. Small spider veins can often be eliminated in one session, though most will require up to three treatments, spaced 8 to 12 weeks apart. Very large spider veins may require even more treatments.

What to do after. If you have a large cluster of spider veins treated on your legs, your doctor may apply bandages to the area and suggest that you elevate your legs for several hours. He may also suggest that you wear compression stockings for the next few days or week or two. If you are predisposed to spider veins or varicose veins, then wearing mild to moderate compression stockings is a good idea anyway. While wearing the stockings might not be pleasant, especially on a hot day, your legs and veins will thank you at bedtime. You should avoid vigorous activity (such as jogging or aerobics) for 24 hours and minimize direct sun exposure to the area for several weeks after treatment. Wear long pants and/or use sunscreen. No sunbathing or tanning booths, unless the treated areas are covered.

Possible side effects and cautions. Side effects for laser treatment of spider veins are rare, but can include slight swelling, redness, or some pain at the treatment site. In rare cases, you might also develop blisters or even scarring. A very rare complication is an outbreak of herpes-like eruptions at the treatment site or in the surrounding area. Those with darker skin may experience temporary pigment changes as a result of the procedure.

Be aware that as the vein is absorbed by the body it will probably undergo color changes. First it may turn black, then within a few days it can lighten, eventually to a light beige; it can then disappear entirely or leave a light beige stain which will lighten with time.

Bear in mind also that there are no guarantees with laser treatment of veins. Although chances are you will have a good cosmetic outcome, some of the veins may still be visible afterwards. Also, it is always possible for the veins to recur and for new ones to develop.

How long until results are apparent. Although the spider veins have been destroyed by the procedure, it may take several weeks or more for the veins to be reabsorbed by the body. A small varicose vein or spider vein may disappear at the time of treatment. It may be erased and gone for good, or it may come back and have to be treated a second or even a third time. If that happens, your doctor may decide to use a different laser or to use injection sclerotherapy. For some reason, some veins respond better to one treatment than the other.

In a condition called "angiomatous matting," the vessels are too small to be seen individually, and can involve multiple layers that stain the skin purple or red and looks like a permanent bruise; in these cases the laser is usually more effective.

In the case of varicose veins, the doctor may request that you return in a few days so that he can lance the vein (it doesn't hurt) and squeeze out some of the material inside. This procedure will speed the resorption of the vein and improve the cosmetic appearance more quickly.

Cost range. $500 to $1,000 per area.

NONLASER TREATMENT FOR SPIDER VEINS

Although lasers offer the quickest and fastest treatment for spider veins and other vascular blemishes, this treatment is not best for everyone, especially those with dark skin. Lasers may be ineffective in treatment of larger varicose veins, which are enlarged and sometimes deformed veins, usually found in the legs. They also don't work as well on larger "starburst" spider veins, again found on the legs space. (Spider veins are in reality a form of varicose veins, involving tiny veins near the surface of the skin.)

INJECTION SCLEROTHERAPY

Injection sclerotherapy is an old and time-tested treatment for varicose veins that can also work for those whose skin type is inappropriate for most laser treatment (although lasers such as the Lyra laser can be used for all skin colors). Injection sclerotherapy involves injecting concentrated saltwater (or detergent) directly into the affected veins, which permanently seals them off. Though the result may be a few weeks of unsightly bruising, the treated vein should eventually be resorbed and disappear completely.

Although the needle used for the injection is small and practically painless of itself, the injected material most commonly used (concentrated salt water) can burn for a minute or two as it travels through the vein. You may also experience cramping in the affected leg. The doctor will advise you to avoid heavy exercise for one or two days after the procedure. Side effects are rare for this procedure.

Cost for sclerotherapy varies, as the charge may be per area treated or per syringe injected, around $200 to $500 per 4 cc syringe. Because small spider veins require more time and effort and a smaller volume of fluid than larger varicose veins, the charge may even be less for the larger varicose veins. The number of syringes used per session will vary depending on the number of veins you need treated. It may take several sessions to get rid of all your unwanted veins.

rosacea

Rosacea is a skin condition of unknown cause in which large portions of the face—usually the cheeks, forehead, and chin—become abnormally red. The red portions of the face may simply appear flushed, or they may be accompanied by the presence of numerous telangiectasia. In some people, acne-like pimples may also appear. In extreme cases, the skin can thicken and become unsightly. In some patients, usually men, the nose can enlarge and become red and deformed ("strawberry nose"). Although rosacea can't be cured, it can be controlled to an extent, by avoiding substances and situations that cause flushing of the face, including heat, exercise, alcohol, hot drinks, spicy foods, chocolate, and rubbing the skin.

The unsightly redness of rosacea can be reduced by the use of lasers targeted to red blemishes. The green Aura laser often gives excellent results with one or two treatments, and also diminishes broken blood vessels on the nose. IPL also works well for rosacea and is considered by many to have superior results. Rosacea-associated pimples, when they occur, are best treated with antibiotics, while an overgrown nose must be corrected by surgery. With laser treatment, first the visible vessels will be individually targeted with a small laser beam, then a larger laser beam will be used (along with simultaneous cooling of the skin) to treat the overall redness. Areas of hyperpigmentation (age spots, liver spots) can be treated at the same time. Ice will often be applied after the treatment, as will a topical steroid, anti-inflammatory cream, or other post-laser cream.

Sun exposure should be limited for a few days after the laser treatment and you should wear a sunscreen (again, this is a good idea any time, especially in those with rosacea). It is common to develop small hives in the affected areas; these can be treated with ice and topical steroids, and will usually resolve in a few days.

skin tags

Skin tags are harmless, soft, wart-like growths that appear more frequently as we grow older. They are usually the color of the skin or light brown, and appear most frequently on the neck, and in the armpits and body folds. They are more common in obese people, but their cause is unknown. Most people find skin tags unsightly; the most common way of getting rid of them is to have a dermatologist freeze them, but they can also be removed with a laser, such as the Aura, or as part of an overall Nlight or Intense Pulsed Light treatment (see chapter 6).

stretch marks

Stretch marks are formed when the skin is stretched to the point that the underlying collagen fibers are damaged. They commonly occur after significant weight gain, especially in a short period of times—pregnancy, for example. Stretch marks can look even worse when the weight then is lost and the underlying skin, which has lost its elasticity, is now excess skin. The whitish-looking striations that result are actually scars where the damaged tissue has healed.

Because the damage has occurred beneath the skin, creams and lotions can't help (though they may make the skin appear smoother). There is some evidence that Retin-A can help fade early stretch marks (those that are still pink or red), but it does nothing for older, pale marks. Exercise can also help a little by firming the musculature beneath the skin, but the white marks will still be visible.

The only thing we have found that truly ameliorates stretch marks is to rebuild the damaged collagen through CoolTouch II laser treatments. A series of four or five treatments at intervals of a few weeks should yield results within a few months, and your skin will continue to look better as new collagen is formed. As a bonus, the texture of the skin will probably improve as well.

creating cheek bones

Models are often said to have "good cheekbones," meaning that their cheekbones are high and prominent, creating lift to their faces and highlighting their eyes. As we get older, our faces tend to droop and the cheekbones recede, becoming less prominent and leading to a flat or hollow look. In the past, the only way to remedy this was to have plastic surgery, including rigid cheek implants.

Today, we can create the illusion of new, prominent cheekbones through a combination of firming the skin (using CoolTouch laser) and selective injectable implants over the area of the cheek ridges. For best results, the injectable implants should be done gradually over multiple sessions. It will take time to achieve the desired results. Unless permanent implants are used (see chapter 5 for various injectable implants and the advantages and disadvantages of each), the results, while long-lasting, will require follow-up injections to be maintained. There is evidence that the injectable implants will stimulate the production of your own collagen and that this will create a more permanent benefit.

sagging or uneven eyebrows

According to Botox pioneers Jean and Alan Carruthers, eighty percent of middle-aged women have eyebrows of noticeably different heights (the difference is usually one or two centimeters, or approximately a third to three quarters of an inch). This is because the muscles on one side of the face have become stronger than on the other over time, and the stronger muscles pull the eyebrow on their side down farther.

Amazingly, most people don't even realize they have an eyebrow discrepancy until it is pointed out to them. Perhaps more obvious, and just as common, is sagging eyebrows. Depending on the facial structure, sagging brows can make you look sad, sleepy, or even angry.

Luckily, uneven and sagging eyebrows can easily be corrected, either as pretreatment for another procedure, or as a stand-alone treatment. For uneven eyebrows, Botox is injected into the muscles above the eyebrow on the side with the higher eyebrow, or below the side with the lower eyebrow, thus weakening those muscles and compensating for the asymmetry. For sagging eyebrows, Botox injections on both sides below the eyebrows will weaken the muscles that pull the brows down, elevating the brows and creating a more wide-awake, brighter look.

too-thin lips

Among the things that happen to all of us as we age is that our lips begin to thin as the natural fat and collagen that keeps them plumped is lost. If your lips were full to begin with, you may not notice this loss, but if you began life with thin lips, the margins around your mouth may seem to disappear.
All of the fillers detailed in chapter 5 have been used for lip implants, but some are more suitable than others.

Be aware that using fillers for lip implantation is a much more uncomfortable procedure than injections for wrinkles. This is because the lips have numerous nerve endings, and also because they move constantly throughout the day, exacerbating any discomfort from the procedure. The good news is that the discomfort only lasts one or two minutes and can be reduced with local anesthetics.

How it works. Your lips are largely mucous tissue, fat and skin, richly supplied with blood and nerves. To augment the lips, the augmentation material is injected in a line beneath the skin. If a material like Gore-Tex, which is supplied in small tubes, is used, a string of material is inserted, usually in two strips per lip.

What to do before. You should meet with your doctor well before the procedure to discuss the look you want to achieve. Some patients, for example, want a soft, sensual, pouty mouth, while others simply want to fill out lips that have thinned with age. Depending on the material to be injected, you may also be given a sample injection at this time to test for allergies. The doctor will probably advise you not to take aspirin or vitamin E, or drink alcohol for up to a week before the procedure (to minimize bleeding or the chance of bruising). You will be asked not to wear lipstick or lip gloss on the day of the procedure.

The procedure. You will be seated in a comfortable reclining medical chair, and the doctor will inject your lip (or lips, if you are having both done) with a local anesthetic. While topical anesthetics can help, an injection of lidocaine inside the mouth (as in a dentist's office) is more effective and might be used. The doctor may have you apply ice to the area to be injected before the injections to decrease both pain and bruising.

When the anesthetic has taken hold, the doctor will inject the filler material, using a tiny needle, along the lip line. The material may cause some pain despite the anesthetic as it is implanted in the lips, but this will last only one or two minutes.

How long it takes. The entire procedure usually takes about 15 minutes per lip.

What to do after. Your doctor will apply ice to your lips and instruct you to continue intermittently icing them for a few hours afterward. Your lips will be slightly sore once the anesthetic wears off, but you should be fine to return to work after your treatment. You should be aware that the lip(s) will be swollen for about a day (sometimes two or three days) after the procedure; while some patients like this appearance of larger lips, most are happier when the swelling is gone. Any bruising will usually last less than a week. Be careful for the first couple of days after the procedure—you probably won't feel like kissing anyone or whistling, but your newly enhanced lips will be worth it in a few days.

It is also possible that the augmentation will not be as full as you had hoped for, because it is always better to under-inject than over-inject. More can always be added, but if you start by injecting too much the swelling will be greater, and if you don't like the enhanced appearance after the swelling is gone, you will have to wait for the material to be absorbed. If you desire additional augmentation, return to the doctor in a couple of weeks for a consultation.

How long until results are apparent. Your lips will be much fuller immediately after the procedure, due in part to swelling from the procedure itself. The swelling should be gone within one to three days, leaving you with your new, full, luscious lips.

How often it needs to be done. The temporary fillers we recommend generally last anywhere from six months to a year or more, but more than one session with incremental augmentation each time is usually the best approach.

Possible side effects and cautions. The procedure will cause your lips to be sore for one to three days afterward. You may also experience some bruising, which usually fades within a week. There is a remote possibility of infection, as with any medical procedure in which the skin is broken, though again this is rare. Be sure to discuss all possible complications with your doctor beforehand.

Cost range. Lip augmentation with injectable fillers, as with wrinkles, depends on the amount of the filler material that must be used and the geographic location where you have the injection performed. The cost *per lip* should range between $300 for collagen to more than $1,500 for some of the newer materials.

tattoo erasure

Do you have a butterfly tattoo on your wrist that doesn't look as good now as it did when you had it applied ten years ago? Do the intertwined snakes on your forearms clash with your current image as an investment banker? If so, you'll be glad to know that some of the lasers we generally employ to ease signs of aging can also erase tattoos.

Tattoos are created by injecting colored pigments (usually mineral compounds) into the middle layers of the skin. The more colors, usually, the more beautiful the tattoo—but also the more difficult it is to remove. Until recently, in fact, it was all but impossible to completely erase these decorative nuisances, and the best that could be done was to scrape and grind the tattoo area, using abrasive substances.

With modern lasers, however, the pigments within a tattoo can be individually targeted and eliminated. Your doctor may need to use more than one laser

New Hope for HIV Patients

Thanks to a number of miraculous new drugs, many people with AIDS are living longer. A side effect of the very drugs that save their lives is that many of these people develop a condition called *lipodystrophy*, in which the fat stores in their body and face disappear, leaving them looking gaunt.

Injectable implants have made it possible for many patients with this condition to return to their former healthy-looking appearance. In most cases, the implants are placed beneath the skin in the hollows of the cheeks, plumping out the face. Although all the materials mentioned in this chapter have been used, one of the most popular implants seems to be New-Fill, because it is relatively long-lasting and doesn't migrate.

to target the different colors. An Alexandrite laser, for example, is often used to remove black, blue, and green pigments, while Nd:YAG-erbium lasers may be used to get rid of almost all colors except green.

Depending on the type, size, and number of colors in the tattoo, it can take up to five treatments or more, approximately a month apart, to completely erase it from your skin. Be aware that tattoo erasure is not painless; many, in fact, describe the pain as equal to that of receiving a tattoo. As treatment progresses, however, there is less pigment available to absorb the laser energy, so the pain decreases. Each treatment should take about ten minutes. A topical anesthetic is usually used, and a soothing dressing is applied afterward. Expect some scabs to form, but scarring is rare, and eventually the skin's normal pigmentation should return.

chapter nine

you and your doctor: having the best rejuvenating experience

Although beauticians also perform many of the treatments and procedures detailed here, we strongly recommend receiving treatment in a medical office or clinic. This is so for multiple reasons. First, only a doctor will have sufficient experience and understanding of all the latest treatments to be able to choose the right treatment or treatment combination for your particular needs. Second, you will have immediate medical attention in the very unlikely event that anything goes wrong; and third, only a medical doctor will be able to prescribe necessary follow-up treatments. Also, and not incidentally, all blemishes are not simply benign. The possibility of cancer must always be kept in mind, and only a doctor has the training to know when to erase with a laser and when to have the "blemish" biopsied.

Partly because of the widespread and growing popularity of Botox, "Botox mills," or discount cosmetic treatment centers, have been springing up across the United States, some of them in shopping malls. In addition to Botox treatments, these clinics may offer other procedures, including microdermabrasion, chemical peels, and some laser treatments.

The problem with these instant clinics is that less-than-fully-qualified medical professionals may staff them. Although you may be tempted to go to a discount rejuvenation clinic, it's simply not worth saving a few dollars—or even a few hundred dollars—if an unsightly appearance is the result. The American Society for Dermatologic Surgery (ASDS) has warned about disastrous results from botched procedures, ranging from severe burns to disfiguring scars. In most cases, these injuries were caused when inexperienced and unaccredited technicians performed the procedures.

We are not saying that you shouldn't visit a cosmetician for very minor procedures, such as superficial peels, or strictly cosmetic treatments such as facials or manicures. But we strongly recommend that you have medical personnel do all other procedures, for all the reasons we mentioned earlier. (Even for these minor procedures, infection can result if qualified personnel do not perform proper sterilization.)

choosing a facility

Before choosing a facility, bear in mind that even if it is staffed by qualified professionals, it still must be clean and use up-to-date equipment. Make sure that any cosmetic facility you enter passes the "look test." If it doesn't look like a clean shop, if you don't look and see the personnel changing the soaking baths between every client, walk out. If you're not sure, ask what precautions they take. If you are not convinced, walk out.

Likewise, be skeptical of testimonials that you see on TV or read in local publications. Testimonials can be misleading or even faked—nothing beats talking to a former client or a practitioner in person. The bottom line is that the best outcome is assured only by making sure that you choose an experienced, licensed practitioner.

With Botox, for example, you need a practitioner who knows not only how much toxin to inject, but precisely where to inject it. If too much Botox is injected, the result could be a bland and expressionless face; too little, and your wrinkles and crow's feet will remain. If the toxin is not injected in the right place, neighboring muscles could be affected, resulting in a drooping eyelid or uneven results, such as one eyebrow being raised much higher than the other.

For other procedures, such as peels and laser treatments, a less experienced practitioner might burn your skin, leaving scars. Improperly administered microdermabrasion can severely scour your face, leading to red, damaged skin. A significant portion of our practice is devoted to repairing mistakes that have been made during prior cosmetic procedures received elsewhere.

Rod P., a semi-retired real estate agent, is one of those lucky people who actually did win the lottery. Although his winnings weren't of the multimillion variety, they left him with enough money to do what he pleased, and what he most wanted was to improve his appearance, which had been ravaged by years of sunbathing.

Nearly fifty now, Rod first came to see us five years ago for foot problems; he became an ongoing patient when he discovered that we could correct the mild disfigurement he'd suffered from four facelifts and other procedures that hadn't turned out as he hoped.

"Take the brow-lifts," he said. "Nobody told me there would be all that scarring." And indeed, when we first saw him, Rod's forehead looked like a battle zone, with depressed scars near the hairline from a surgical lift and a ridge near the midline from an implant that failed to smooth out heavy furrows.

Among his other procedures were a cheekbone implant that had migrated, leaving a hard ridge on each side of his face below his eyes, and a lip implant that had hardened.

"All I wanted was to look better," Rod explained. "I thought it would be simple, but it turned out it wasn't."

Using many of the techniques we've mentioned earlier in this book, we managed to restore Rod's native good looks. For the depressed scars and ridge on his forehead, we used injectable implants to even out the surface of the skin. The eye problem was a little more problematic, but using a combination of Botox and injectable implants, we managed to even out that area too, which saved Rod from having to have another surgery to remove the migrated transplant.

We also used the CoolTouch laser on the more weathered-looking parts of Rod's face. He was very pleased with the results as his skin began to plump up and look younger within a few weeks. These days, Rod looks at least fifteen years younger than his age, with smooth, glowing skin, a full, sensuous mouth (thanks to new implants), and a toned and muscular body from working out several times a week.

finding the right doctor

Since the treatments and procedures discussed in this book don't involve surgery, you needn't necessarily go to a plastic surgeon. Many plastic surgeons do provide the medical but less radical treatments we detail, as do most dermatologists and many other practitioners of different specialties. Whatever sort of physician you choose, be certain that he or she is accredited both by the local medical society and his or her specialty. If you are receiving laser treatments, one useful guide is if your doctor is a Diplomate of the American Society of Lasers in Medicine and Surgery. For information on checking out your doctor's credentials, see the box on page 106 and the web sites in Appendix B.

One of the best ways to find a good doctor is to ask around. Perhaps your family doctor can recommend someone. If you have friends who've had cosmetic work done, ask them to tell you about their experience and whether they would recommend their doctor. Other places to get tips are beauty parlors and health clubs. Nearly everyone knows someone who's had at least one procedure, even if it's only a simple Botox injection.

In addition to accreditation, your doctor must have the experience and artistry to recommend and perform the best treatments for you as an individual. Not every doctor has an eye for beauty. While he or she may be able to competently inject implants or Botox, or to wield the CoolTouch laser, it's important to work with a doctor who can envision your entire face as it is now and as it will look after the treatments.

It's a Matter of Health

Seeking a qualified physician to perform your anti-aging treatments can mean much more than a better aesthetic outcome, resulting in younger-looking skin. It can also have implications for your long-term health.

Remember that anti-aging treatments should be regarded as medical treatments above all. Only a physician is qualified to distinguish between blemishes that can be treated with lasers and suspicious blemishes which should be biopsied. Although a laser treatment may eliminate the appearance of a seemingly harmless red or brown bump, if that spot was actually an early cancer, the cancer may continue to spread. For more on suspicious bumps and spots, see page 000.

You shouldn't assume, just because a doctor has a fancy, attractively decorated office, that he or she is qualified and experienced. In addition to the surroundings, it's important to examine the general atmosphere of a prospective doctor's offices. Before making a decision, visit the office to see if you are well treated and feel comfortable. Bear in mind that many of the procedures we recommend will need to be repeated from time to time, so you should not patronize a doctor with whom you don't feel comfortable or whose staff is rude. Be sure to check out in advance the costs of any procedures you will receive. Remember that prices vary somewhat in different areas of the country and from office to office.

Throughout this book, we offer guidelines to costs for most procedures, but for the latest up-to-date information, check the Internet (see Appendix B for links). Also, remember that in rejuvenation treatments, as with so many other areas in life, you get what you pay for. This is definitely not the place to cut corners.

WHAT TO LOOK FOR IN A DOCTOR

- **Make sure that your first interview is with a qualified physician, not a technician or assistant**, and that staff members are experienced and properly trained. Don't be afraid to ask; if you don't receive satisfactory answers, go elsewhere for your treatments.

    Although it may sound like superfluous advice, it's important for you to have realistic expectations. Each of the products and procedures detailed in this book can create a noticeable and sometimes profound difference in your appearance, but none of them will make you nineteen again, and none will transform you into a movie star or supermodel.

- **No matter what your doctor's specialty, be certain that he or she has ample experience performing the procedure you are contemplating.** It's best to choose someone with experience in a wide variety of cosmetic techniques, because only someone with that background can determine which of several treatments are right for you, or if you would get better results by combining two or more procedures. If a carpenter only has a hammer, everything might look like a nail; you want a carpenter with a complete tool box.

HOW TO EVALUATE A DOCTOR

As we stressed in an earlier chapter, good communication between doctor and patient is the key to a successful outcome in any medical procedures. When you meet with your physician for the first time, don't hesitate to share any of your concerns. Although you may feel nervous asking the doctor about his or her credentials and experience, a reputable physician will readily supply this information and any other that's directly relevant to your planned procedure.

The physician should also have a prepared sheet explaining what to do before the procedure (drugs and pills to avoid, whether you should stay out of the sun) and what to expect after the procedure (pain, swelling, restrictions on activity, medications to take or avoid). Even if he gives you a printout, the doctor should also offer detailed instructions on pre- and post-procedure care.

QUESTIONS TO ASK

In addition to the obvious questions about costs and financing, you might ask to see before and after photos or videotapes of patients who have had the same procedure you are considering. Other questions you may want to ask include:

- **Are my desired results realistic? If not, what is the best outcome I can hope for?** Beware of doctors who "promise the moon." While nearly everyone will benefit from the various procedures we describe in this book, the degree of improvement in your appearance will depend on a number of factors, including your age, type of skin, degree of sun damage, and underlying muscular structure. If you currently look like Yoda, even the most skilled physician can't make you into Barbie.
- **Are there other procedures that might give me a better result than the one I have in mind?** As we've stressed throughout this book, no one procedure alone can do everything. For many problems, such as old acne scars or deep lines in the skin, injectable fillers are great, but they can't do a thing for skin discolorations. Botox can relax wrinkles, but doesn't help scars. (An exception might be when there is asymmetrical muscle activity caused by a scar.) Microdermabrasion can give your skin a much smoother and pleasing appearance, but it doesn't reduce brow furrows. Your physician should give you a detailed list of treatments available and what you can expect from each. She or he should also offer alternative treatments if they are more appropriate.

- **How many times have you performed this particular procedure? How long have you been doing this procedure?** If your doctor is fully qualified, she won't mind giving you a candid answer to these questions.
- **How many of your patients have had complications from this procedure?** Again, a competent and qualified doctor will have no qualms about sharing this information.
- **Has this laser system been approved specifically for someone with my skin type, hair color, and complexion? Is it specifically approved for use on the part of my body that I want treated?** There are a growing number of medical lasers available, and not all are appropriate for all treatments or all patients. Your doctor should be prepared to explain the exact prescribed uses of the laser he intends to use on your treatment.
- **Can I contact some of your previous patients?** Don't be afraid to ask to speak to other patients, and when you do, ask for their candid appraisal, both of the procedure and their interaction with the doctor.
- **If I'm not pleased with the outcome, will you repeat or correct the treatment without charging me extra?** Some doctors will ask you to return approximately two weeks after your treatment for a follow-up visit, at which time any additional needed treatment can be done. If the original results were unsatisfactory, and depending upon the reason why, a reputable doctor should be willing to touch up the treatment as necessary for no extra charge.

CAUTIONS

While the majority of doctors are ethical and dedicated to their patients' welfare, there are bad apples in every bunch, including some who may try to make an extra profit by cutting corners—for instance, by using an overly diluted or stale preparation of Botox. If a doctor charges you much less than the going rate for any procedure, it's possible that he is cutting corners in some way or is very inexperienced and quickly trying to build up a patient base.

Beware of doctors who:

- Will not show you their certification
- Tell you that one procedure will solve all of your cosmetic problems
- Refuse to let you speak to previous patients
- Charge much less than the going rate
- Are too rushed to give you adequate time for consultation before your procedure

How to Check a Doctor's Credentials

One good way to find a qualified doctor is to check out your local medical societies or use one of the many physician locator services on the Internet (see Appendix B for URLs).

To find out if your doctor is on the up-and-up, you can also check if he is listed with the American Board of Medical Specialties (ABMS), an organization of 24 approved medical specialty boards. The organization's web site (listed in Appendix B) offers a database of physicians who have completed an approved training program and evaluation process assessing their ability to provide quality care in the given specialty.

Keep in mind that the field of minimally and non-invasive cosmetic medicine is in its infancy and therefore in constant change. A board-certified dermatologist or plastic surgeon might have extensive experience and expertise with lasers, Botox, and other cosmetic procedures--or he might not. A doctor who is a specialist, but not a dermatologist or plastic surgeon, might have gained extensive experience, knowledge, and abilities in the field of minimally invasive cosmetic medicine and be your best choice. The only way to find out is to ask.

You can also check your state licensing board to make certain that your physician's medical license is up-to-date. Most state medical licensing boards can also be found on the Internet. Just enter [Your state] Board of Medical Examiners in a search engine.

chapter ten

non-medical ways to beautify your skin

I n the bad old days of just a decade or two ago, the promises made by cosmetic companies were just that—promises, as empty as the tubes and bottles customers discarded in their vain search for a youthful appearance. Thanks to a number of scientific breakthroughs, many over-the-counter products now actually do what they promise, not only making your skin appear younger and fresher, but actually rejuvenating it.

Although medical solutions (CoolTouch laser, Botox, microdermabrasion, Renova) are still the fastest routes to a rejuvenated appearance, you needn't go to a doctor's office to begin reversing the aging process in your skin. Many of these products will give you similar results (though not so quickly and dramatically as medical treatments). There are also a number of products that can (and should) be used to enhance and protect the results obtained with medical procedures.

107

what your skin needs to look its best

The prescription and the over-the-counter products detailed in this book can all help you look younger. But in addition to these special treatments, for your complexion to look its best, you must give it a minimal amount of routine care.

Wash. There are two important watchwords for your face: cleanliness and moisture. Not only is clean skin healthy, it looks better. Washing twice daily helps prevent clogged pores and helps clear away the dead cells on the outer layer of your skin. We recommend using a mild non-soap product, such as Cetaphil, available in drugstores. Another good cleanser is Staraphil Lotion.

Moisturize. Moisturizing can be accomplished with only one substance: water. All the potions and lotions you see advertised for moisturizing the skin do one of two things: they attract moisture to the skin or they keep moisture within your skin from evaporating. When we're young, the natural oils on the skin do a good job of protecting our natural moisture. However, oil production declines with age, which is why it's necessary to replace it.

Protect. Once your face is clean and dry, you need to apply something to protect it. During the day, a moisturizing cream or lotion with an SPF of at least 15 is a must. (See "Don't Forget the Sunscreen!," page 137). If you use Renova, apply it alone before bedtime. If you are using Kinerase, alpha-hydroxy, or retinol-based products, they can be used on your non-Renova nights, and should go on before your moisturizer.

choosing the right products

Although they may be in prettier bottles and have a better texture than the creams and lotions our mothers and grandmothers used, basic creams and lotions haven't changed much since early in the last century. It's another story, however, for the new ingredients added to these basic potions.

For the first time in cosmetic history, over-the-counter "wrinkle creams" can actually help to reduce and prevent wrinkles, as well as help restore firmness, smooth texture, and restore a more blemish-free appearance to skin. Also known as "cosmeceuticals," for their restorative properties, these treatments and cosmetics have revolutionized the cosmetics counter. Though none of the products detailed in this chapter will give results as dramatic as the prescription products and the medical procedures described earlier in the book, the truth is that many of them can and will make a visible difference in your appearance, provided you buy top of the line products and apply them as directed.

Following is a guide to what is currently available without prescription. Be aware that many of these products are quite pricey—as expensive as prescription preparations or the equivalent medical procedure. Before we begin, with so many products out there, it's hard to know which to choose.

CREAMS VERSUS LOTIONS VERSUS OINTMENTS

Creams, lotions, even ointments, what are the differences? Which is best for you? The lighter preparations are creams and lotions, which, despite what the cosmetic ads say, are simply a mixture of oil and water, along with a number of other ingredients such as scents, stabilizers, and preservatives. Lotions and creams may also be used to deliver other substances that can affect your skin, such as Kinerase or vitamin C.

- Lotions have relatively more water than creams and feel liquid.
- Creams have a more solid consistency.
- Ointments are also a mixture of oil and water, but have a heavier concentration of oil and feel greasy to the touch. Ointments are the best moisturizers for very dry skin or for all types of skin in extreme weather conditions.

As to which sort of preparation to choose, that depends in part on your age, the time of year, and the part of the country in which you live. The oilier your skin, the lighter the product you should use. Most types of skin, except very oily, should avoid products that contain alcohols, which can be drying.

ALPHA-HYDROXY AND GLYCOLIC ACID PRODUCTS

You may recall that in chapter 3 we talked about prescription-strength alpha-hydroxy and glycolic acid peels and lotions. All of these products are made from alpha-hydroxy acids, which are naturally occuring acids found in fruits, sugar cane, and milk. Glycolic acids, among the most widely used, are alpha-hydroxy acids that are made from sugar cane.

It's interesting that the most common use of alpha-hydroxy acids is in over-the-counter skincare products, which contain a lesser concentration of the acids than prescription products. Can such relatively weak potions actually make a difference in the way your skin looks? Surprisingly, the answer is yes—provided that you know what you're looking for, buy established brands, and follow the manufacturer's directions.

The key to a product's effectiveness is in its percentage of glycolic or alpha-hydroxy acid. Most over-the-counter products contain acids in the range of 3 to 5 percent. Although the numbers aren't exact, many experts believe that concentrations below 8 percent are worthless. Studies of products with alpha-hydroxy acid concentrations of 8 to 15 percent do report definite improvement—though minor—in wrinkles and skin smoothness.

Prescription-strength AHA (alpha-hydroxy acid) and glycolic acid creams and lotions typically contain a 15 to 20 percent concentration (while prescription-strength peels, applied in a doctor's office, contain an even higher percentage (20%-70% glycolic acid). Preparations of this strength have been shown in medical tests to improve skin texture, reduce fine lines and wrinkles, and improve acne. Because they are much stronger than over-the-counter products they are more likely to cause skin irritation, redness, and peeling. Glycolic acid can even cause skin color darkening (especially in people of color), so it should only be used under a doctor's supervision.

CHOOSING EFFECTIVE AHA PRODUCTS

So how do you choose truly effective over-the-counter fruit-acid skin products? We recommend looking for brands with a concentration in the high end of the 8 to 15 percent range, though you should be aware that the higher the percentage of active ingredient, the more likely a product is to cause skin irritation. Another problem is that over-the-counter products with higher amounts of acid typically contain buffering agents to prevent irritation and peeling, which make the active ingredient less effective.

Be aware that even over-the-counter AHA and glycolic acid products can increase sensitivity to the sun, so you should always use them in conjunction with a sunscreen SPF 15 or higher. Also, as with the prescription-strength products, these products' effects on your skin last only as long as you use them. As soon as you quit using the product, your skin will gradually return to its former condition.

How they work. Like many of the new rejuvenating products, alpha-hydroxy acids work by accelerating sloughing of the outer layers of skin. This mildly damages your skin in such a way that cell replenishment is increased. They also may affect the production of new cells beneath the skin and even mildly stimulate collagen renewal.

How to use alpha-hydroxy acids. Be sure to read the directions on the package, but in general alpha and glycolic acid products should be applied daily to a clean face, then followed with sunscreen (if applied during the day). If you notice stinging, redness, or peeling, reduce use to every other day for a week or two. If you continue to experience irritation, try a different brand or a milder product, such as one containing beta-hydroxy acid (see below).

Possible side effects and cautions. When they are used properly, there are very few side effects from over-the-counter alpha-hydroxy acid products. Mild stinging, peeling, or redness are the most common, and they will disappear if you discontinue using the product.

How long until results are apparent. Depending on how well you have taken care of your skin in the past, you should start to notice a difference within a very few weeks. Many people find their skin looks and feels smoother, fine wrinkles and age spots begin to fade, and the pores appear smaller.

BETA-HYDROXY ACID PRODUCTS

Among the growing number of miracle ingredients added to cosmetic products are BHAs (beta-hydroxy acids), which, like alpha-hydroxy acids, occur naturally. The most commonly used beta-hydroxy acid is salicylic acid, which is derived from the bark of the willow tree and is closely related to aspirin. Beta-hydroxy acids are often combined with alpha-hydroxy acids in exfoliating preparations.

Beta-hydroxy acids are similar in effect to alpha-hydroxy acids; they exfoliate the top layers of skin, resulting in a smoother and clearer complexion. They also minimize the appearance of fine lines and wrinkles. Beta-hydroxy acids are in general less irritating to the skin than alpha-hydroxy and glycolic acids, and are often combined with alpha-hydroxy acids in the same products.

The FDA has determined that beta-hyroxy acids, like retinols and alpha-hydroxys, increase sensitivity to the sun and should always be used in conjunction with a sunscreen, SPF 15 or higher.

Use of beta-hydroxy acid products is similar to that of alpha-hydroxy acid and glycolic acid products.

MILD MASKS AND PEELS

There are a number of superficial masks and peels using alpha-hydroxy or gly-colic acids that you can safely apply at home. Although the results aren't per-manent, peels exfoliate the dead, dull skin cells on the surface of the epidermis, giving you a brighter and clearer complexion. As with all the products men-tioned in this chapter, superficial peels produce immediately visible results, but not as intense as those obtained with prescription products or those applied by a doctor or cosmetician.

How they work. Home-use masks and peels loosen dead skin cells from the surface of the skin (exfoliating them), revealing a smoother and clearer complex-ion and speeding up the skin's natural cell turnover process. Because they contain mild acids, these products may sting or tingle when you apply them.

How to use them. Follow the instructions on the label. Most products are best used once or twice a week; overuse can cause your skin to become irritat-ed and to peel.

Possible side effects and cautions. As with any fruit-acid products, there's always a chance of irritation or peeling. Also, your skin may become sen-sitized to the sun, so be religious in your use of sun protection. Use SPF 15 or higher, and reapply often, especially if you sweat or go swimming.

How long until results are apparent. The great thing about over-the-counter masks and peels is that your skin will look noticeably clearer and brighter immediately; with continued use, it will look even better.

some recommended brands of over-the-counter AHA, BHA, and glycolic acid skin preparations

There are literally hundreds of brands and thousands of preparations. The fol-lowing list is by no means intended to be exhaustive, but to serve, rather, as a guideline. In general, we recommend buying products from established, rep-utable companies. As a rule, you can trust any product your doctor sells through his office or clinic. Note that we also offer our own exclusive brand of products, as do other doctors and spas, that offer protection and enhancement from head to toe. (See Appendix B.)

Brands of peels, lotions, masks, and scrubs available in department stores, drugstores, and through sales representatives:

- Avon Anew
- Neutrogena
- ROC
- Clinique

RETINOL

Retinol, a vitamin-A derivative, is a precursor to tretinoin, the prescription product used to combat acne and as the active ingredient in the popular prescription cream Renova. Like Renova, retinol creams are said to make skin smoother and firmer, while reducing surface blemishes. In theory, retinol is absorbed into the skin, where it is converted to active tretinoin. However, retinol is five times weaker than tretinoin, and will not work as effectively nor as quickly as the prescription cream.

Nevertheless, millions of satisfied customers have happily used retinol products to make their skins smoother and younger looking. According to Rachel Grossman and Stanley Shapiro, Director of Medical Affairs and Director of Preclinical Research, respectively, for Johnson & Johnson, retinol cannot be considered a direct substitute for the stronger prescription product. In an interview given to Paula Begoun on the CosmeticsCop web site, Grossman and Shapiro explain that retinol should be considered primarily by people whose skin is too sensitive to tolerate the active ingredient in Renova.

How to use. When buying retinol products, get the strongest preparation you can find among established brands. The highest strength commonly sold in over-the-counter products ranges from 0.03% to 0.15% retinol. Retinol may be weaker than tretinoin, the active ingredient in Renova, but it should still be treated with caution. Before applying, first wash your face and wait for it to dry. Instructions often recommend waiting fifteen minutes to half an hour, because applying retinol to a damp face can increase the chances for irritation. When your face is dry, apply a small amount (the instructions often recommend the size of a pea) to your face and neck and gently rub it in with your fingertips. As with Retinol, more is *not* better here, and is only more likely to irritate your skin.

Note: be sure to wash your hands when you have finished, and also take care to keep the product out of your eyes.

The labels on most over-the-counter retinol products recommend that the product be applied before bedtime, and not be used at the same time as any other product. It's best to begin every other night (or even less frequently if you have very sensitive skin) and then increase the frequency until you are using the over-the-counter retinol five to seven nights a week. If you notice any irritation or peeling, cut back on usage until your skin has become accustomed to the retinol and the irritation has disappeared.

Possible side effects and cautions. Like tretinoin, retinol sensitizes your skin to sunlight, so you should always wear a sunscreen of SPF 15 or higher and stay out of the sun as much as possible (see chapter 12 for more sun-avoidance tips). Also, although retinol is closely related to tretinoin, it can actually stimulate oil production and cause acne. In addition, some users find that it irritates their skin much as Renova does, causing redness, stinging, itching, or peeling. If you notice any of those symptoms, decrease or stop use immediately.

If you are pregnant, you should *not* use a retinol product, no matter how small the percentage of retinol, because of the remote possibility that it might cause birth defects.

How long until results are apparent. You'll need to use a retinol product for at least three weeks before you begin to notice a change in your skin. The results—smoother, clearer, more finely textured skin—should continue to improve for several months as long as you continue to use the product.

Cost range. Retinol products tend to be pricey, especially when compared to Renova, which is fairly economical in the small amounts used. In general, prices range from as little as around $20 for up to five ounces to nearly $40 for half an ounce. Always check the label, and remember that the percentage of the active ingredient is more important than fancy packaging. Brands available in doctors' offices (or over the Internet) are generally more expensive, but usually contain a higher percentage of retinol.

Brands available in doctors' offices and on the Internet:

- M.D. Forté
- Afirm

Brands available in department stores, drugstores, and through sales representatives:

- ROC
- Avon Anew
- Afirm
- Cetaphil
- Neutrogena

KINERASE (FURFURYLADENINE)

A new product that promises to perform as well as or even better than Renova is Kinerase (another product name is Kinetin), which is derived from a growth factor in plants. This compound, furfuryladenine, retards aging in plants (cut leaves treated with furfuryladenine stay green, while untreated leaves turn brown).

Though not as widely studied as Renova, Kinerase appears to provide some of the same benefits on human skin. Unlike Renova, Kinerase is designed to be applied to the neck, shoulders, chest, and hands, as well as the face. It is considered safe for pregnant and lactating women, and works well for those with sensitive skin.

Kinerase is an excellent moisturizer, actually improving the ability of the skin to retain moisture. Katya, our patient from New Mexico who applied Renova each night to prevent or at least slow down further aging changes in her skin, also used Kinerase during the day. "It's so dry out in the desert where I do most of my work," she said. "Even with the Renova, I tend to look parched. Kinerase seems to make a big difference. I put it on first, then my sun screen, and my skin looks much smoother and more youthful."

How it works. Scientists aren't quite sure how Kinerase works, but it has been shown to be a powerful antioxidant, which probably accounts for at least some of its effects. In tests, many people who have used it are as satisfied or more satisfied than those who use Renova. Because Kinerase also acts as a moisturizer, it immediately lessens the appearance of fine lines and wrinkles, and leaves skin feeling smoother and softer.

Kinerase feels like any other lotion going on. There should be no burning or stinging, as there sometimes is with Renova and glycolic acid products. Kinerase is available in both lotion and cream form, depending on your needs.

How to apply. You should apply Kinerase twice a day. First, wash your face with a mild soap or cleanser and allow your skin to dry, then apply a dime-size amount to your fingertips and gently rub it on your face and neck. Because Kinerase isn't affected by other chemicals, you can apply other lotions or creams, including makeup and sunscreen, directly over it. You can even use it in conjunction with other treatments, such as alpha-hydroxy creams or Renova, as long as you use the products at different times of the day.

Possible side effects and cautions. Unlike Renova, Kinerase has few if any side effects. In a study, patients who used it had no problem with redness, flaking, or burning. Even better, Kinerase doesn't increase susceptibility to sun exposure.

How long until results are apparent. Since Kinerase is a very good moisturizer, you may notice an improvement in your skin as soon as you begin using it. A more visible and general improvement may take a few weeks to up to six months.

Cost range. A small tube of Kinerase (1.4 ounces), costs from around $43 to $55, and should last about two months. The larger size (3.8 ounces) is more economical, costing from $72 to $90 or more. At present, Kinerase is available only on the Internet and through doctors' offices. Check the Internet for specials; the cost for Kinerase, like the cost for many other specialty cosmetic products, can vary widely from site to site. (It is also available at our web site, listed in Appendix B.)

COPPER PEPTIDES

Copper, which is the third-most abundant trace mineral in the human body, is found in most tissues, especially in blood and connective tissue (such as collagen). It has been proven essential for the strength and flexibility of skin, and is a major factor in wound healing. In fact, copper-containing preparations are often used after deep peels to help speed the skin's healing process.

When copper-peptide preparations are applied to the skin, small amounts of the active ingredient (prezatide copper acetate, which is hydrolyzed soy protein chelated to copper chloride) penetrate the skin, where it has been shown to stimulate the growth of collagen, leading to wrinkle reduction and improved skin firmness. Copper is also said to help improve skin blotchiness, through stimulating the outer skin's regeneration process. The minute amount of copper in cosmetic preparations is considered safe, and does not raise blood levels of copper.

How to use. Although directions for use of copper preparations will differ somewhat depending on the manufacturer and the exact formula, the following tips will serve as a general guide for most products.

Apply a small amount of the copper-peptide preparation once or twice a day. Most manufacturers suggest that you start with a very small amount every other day and then increase the amount and frequency as your skin becomes accustomed to it. Some people with very sensitive skin may continue to experience irritation or inflammation; if that is the case, try another copper-peptide formula. If you are also using a vitamin C preparation, alternate it with the copper-peptides every other morning, because there is some evidence that vitamin C can inactivate copper when they are used together topically.

Possible side effects and cautions. Not all copper peptides are good for your skin. Though not dangerous, some copper preparations are ineffective. To be sure you are using a safe and effective product, buy copper preparations only from well-known manufacturers. If in doubt, ask your dermatologist for a recommendation.

How long until results are apparent. It may take three to four months of frequent use to see an improvement in your skin.

Cost range. Copper-peptide preparations vary widely in price. For example, half an ounce of Neutrogena eye cream is $19; the same amount from Neova is $39; while a similar bottle from Skin Biology costs $24. Shop around and check the Internet before you buy.

Brands available in doctors' offices and on the Internet:

• Neova (Procyte), a line of fragrance-free products sold only through physicians
• Protect & Restore (Skin Biology)

Brands available in department stores, drugstores, and through sales representatives:

• Visibly Firm (Neutrogena)

decoding the alphabet soup of vitamin products

Vitamins no longer come only in pill form. Instead they are now among the most touted ingredients in prescription and over-the-counter skin care products. When evaluating these products, there are two main considerations: is the vitamin or other nutrient truly effective, and is it delivered to the skin in a way that will enable it to work?

The most important of the vitamins and other nutrients used for skin care are those classed as antioxidants. Antioxidants have become buzzwords in the last few years, their benefits proclaimed in everything from multivitamins to shampoos. The reason for their great press is that antioxidants are natural compounds that have the ability to prevent and even repair some of the damage done to the body by free radicals, destructive molecules that can be created by many things including ultraviolet light (sunlight, tanning beds), pollution, or even normal body metabolism.

Though free radicals are extremely short-lived, they cause damage quickly, breaking down collagen and diminishing the skin's firmness and texture. Antioxidants help to inactivate free radicals before they can do their damage. Topical antioxidants are more effective in preventing or even helping to reverse some of this damage in the skin than those taken orally, though oral antioxidants are useful for the rest of the body. It helps to apply topical antioxidants to the sun-exposed portions of your skin daily, but keep in mind that these are not a substitute for limiting sun exposure and wearing a sunscreen.

It may seem hard to believe that antioxidants, which are basically nutritional substances, can actually work their magic inside the skin. Yet with one of these substances, vitamin A, the evidence is incontrovertible that it changes the very structure of the skin. Tretinoin, the active ingredient in Retin-A and Renova, is basically a derivative of vitamin A, as is retinol, the over-the-counter version (see chapter 3).

With other vitamins, however, the evidence is somewhat less clear-cut. According to Dr. Karen A. Burke, speaking at the 2002 meeting of the American Academy of Dermatology, most over-the-counter preparations don't contain enough antioxidants to have any effect, or they are poorly absorbed by the skin. However, she mentions three antioxidants in particular that have been proven to prevent or even reverse the signs of aging when applied to the skin: selenium, vitamin E, and vitamin C.

118

Although high doses of some antioxidants (such as vitamin A) can be toxic when taken orally, there's no evidence of any danger when these antioxidants are applied to the skin. Two antioxidants that do work when applied topically are vitamins C and E. It's important to bear in mind that antioxidants do not work alone; they are effective only in concert with other antioxidants and other essential nutrients, such as zinc. For recommendations on supplements, see chapter 18.

> **Caution:** unlike many cosmetic products, antioxidant creams have a comparatively short shelf life. Be sure to read labels and don't use products that have passed their expiration date.

VITAMIN C

There is no longer controversy over the protective powers of relatively large doses of vitamin C taken internally. Though it is not yet so well-known, vitamin C is also very effective as a topical cream or lotion, and has been shown in numerous studies to actually help repair broken collagen in that form. Vitamin C is the most abundant antioxidant found naturally in the skin, where it also plays a role in preventing pre-cancers from turning into cancers.

Vitamin C is depleted whenever the skin is exposed to the sun, pollution, or smoking; even minimal ultraviolet exposure can decrease the vitamin C levels in the skin by 30 percent, while exposure to the ozone of city pollution can decrease the level by 55 percent.

It seems obvious that one of the most important things you can do for your skin is to replace its hard-working vitamin C. It might be tempting to think you can just increase your consumption of vitamin C pills, and we certainly do recommend taking vitamin C daily. However, the truth is that excess vitamin C is simply eliminated from the body in the urine; little of it gets to the skin in a sufficient concentration needed for prevention and rejuvenation. So, in addition to taking vitamin C orally (see chapter 18 for details), use a good, prescription-strength cream or lotion to help prevent and repair damage inside your skin and stimulate the formation of new collagen.

Properly formulated vitamin C creams and lotions can not only help to repair oxidative damage, they help prevent more of it from occurring. Regular use of a good vitamin C product can improve the overall tone and texture of your skin, making it look smoother, firmer, and less lined. In addition to the benefits already named, as a bonus, vitamin C can help repair sun damage by neutralizing free radicals before they can cause oxidation damage to your skin.

Note: Vitamin C is not a sunscreen; even if you use a good topical vitamin C product, don't go out in the sun without the addition of a good SPF 30 sunscreen.

We don't recommend using just any vitamin C product. The vitamin C pills you take—the most common form of the nutrient—are primarily L-ascorbic acid, which is the most biologically active form, but which unfortunately breaks down rapidly when exposed to oxygen. In order for the vitamin to penetrate your skin and begin to work its magic, the L-ascorbic acid first needs to be stabilized, and at a high enough concentration to affect your skin. It also needs to be formulated with a low pH (acid-base balance) of 3.5 or less.

Some companies use a different, less effective form of vitamin C, or include an ineffectively low concentration of L-ascorbic acid.

How to use. For best results, use your vitamin C preparation daily, preferably in the morning. If you are also using a product containing copper, you should alternate it with the vitamin C, because there is evidence that vitamin C can inactivate copper. Vitamin C can be applied at any time of day, but if you use it in the morning, be sure to apply the vitamin C preparation before your sunscreen and makeup. If you use it in the evening, we recommend that you apply a good moisturizer after the vitamin C.

Possible side effects and problems. Vitamin C is completely safe for your skin. Rarely, you may notice mild dryness or flaking, which can be easily handled with a moisturizer.

How long until results are apparent. Although you may notice some softening and smoothing of your skin within a few weeks, it generally takes two to three months for lines and wrinkles to noticeably diminish. A maximum effect will occur at about six months.

Recommended vitamin C products. Buy only a very good, established brand of vitamin C with a concentration of at least 10 percent L-ascorbic acid (see recommendations below). Up to 20 percent concentration is better, but it may be hard on sensitive skin, or skin affected by rosacea. The product should also be stabilized and formulated with a low pH so it will be absorbed into your skin.

The following list is not meant to be exhaustive. These are products that appear to be effective. At present they are available only through physicians and the Internet:

- **Neova-C Protection Crème.** Contains 10 percent L-ascorbic acid. Made by Procyte and available through physicians and the Internet.
- **Cellex-C.** Contains 10 percent L-ascorbic acid with a pH of 2.8, along with zinc and tyrosine, co-factors that enhance its activity. Made by Cellex-C and available through the Internet.
- **SkinC Skin Firming Cream.** Contains 10 percent L-ascorbic acid. Made by SkinCeuticals, Inc. Available only through physicians. SkinCeuticals also makes the Primacy line, which contains a higher concentration of L-ascorbic acid,
- **Institute Beauté brand.** 15 percent L-ascorbic acid, available as a serum or cream.

VITAMIN E

Like vitamin C, vitamin E is an important antioxidant. Whereas vitamin C works primarily in the watery part of tissue, vitamin E is most effective in fatty tissues, such as cell membranes. It is essential for tissue repair and healing and helps prevent blood clots.

Vitamin E ointment has long been used to help speed healing of wounds and diminish scars. Numerous studies have shown that taking vitamin E regularly helps protect against many diseases of aging. Now vitamin E has become one of the hot new ingredients in skin care.

Unfortunately, like vitamin C, topical vitamin E has to be in a specific form to be effective. The predominant form of vitamin E found in tissues is *alpha-tocopherol*, which has the greatest biological activity of all forms of vitamin E. Other names used for this form of vitamin E are: mixed tocopherols, d-alpha tocopherol, and DL-alpha tocopherol.

Tocopherol is the only form of vitamin E that your body can use. *Other, non-tocopherol, forms of vitamin E will not work as antioxidants.* Nevertheless, a number of cosmetic companies use these derivatives of vitamin E, sometimes claiming antioxidant properties. The way to spot derivatives of vitamin E is to carefully read the ingredients list. If the name for the vitamin E ends in "tocopherol," as with the variants listed above, then it is biologically active.

The nonactive derivatives of vitamin E are labeled "tocopheryl," followed by another word, typically acetate, linoleate, nicotinate, or succinate. Thus, any product that contains such ingredients as "D-alpha tocopheryl nicotinate" or "tocopheryl acetate" may be fine as a moisturizer (the vitamin E derivatives are good emollients), but will not repair free radical damage or protect against sun damage.

How it works. Vitamin E works best in combination with other substances, including vitamin C and zinc, so it is often packaged in a combination product. Its strongest property is its antioxidant capabilities. Studies have shown that not only does it protect against (and repair) damage from free radicals, it also can protect against and repair damage caused by UVB (ultraviolet B) sunlight. It also promotes healing and may help prevent age spots.

Vitamin E creams can be applied daily, and used with other products, except for Renova, which should be applied alone. So if you are also using Renova, apply vitamin E at a different time of day.

Possible side effects. Rarely, topical Vitamin E preparations can cause contact dermatitis and itching, sometimes severe.

Recommended vitamin E products. The following list is not meant to be exhaustive. These are products that appear to be effective. Most are available only through physicians.

There are few effective brands of vitamin E and vitamin E and C combination creams. When searching for an effective product, remember to check the ingredients list according to the guidelines we've recommended in this chapter. Among the effective creams we can recommend are:

- **Primacy Face Cream (Skinceuticals).** This product is soy-based, because soy can act as an estrogen on aging skin, stimulating production of hyaluronate and collagen. It also contains silimaryn, a powerful antioxidant derived from milk thistle, and 3 percent vitamin E (alpha tocopherol).
- **Primacy C & E Serum (Skinceuticals).** This product contains 15 percent L-ascorbic acid and 2 percent alpha tocopherol.

Cost range. Topical vitamin products tend to be extremely pricey, which makes it even more important to carefully check the ingredients lists and make sure you are getting what you are paying for—check the Internet for best prices. As an example, a half-ounce jar of Cellex-C high-potency eye gel can cost anywhere from $36 to $46; Skinceuticals' 50 ml SkinC Skin Firming

Cream is available at prices ranging from $53 to $85. Similar spreads exist for vitamin E and combination creams.

skin lighteners

Long before alpha-hydroxy acids and Kinerase hit the market, people with sun damage used various skin lighteners to fade sun-caused age spots. The majority of skin-lightening products contain 2 percent hydroquinone, which prevents melanin, the skin's dark pigment, from forming. Although we believe that equally good or better results can be obtained from using AHA and glycolic acid products, or having microdermabrasion, you may want to try a lightening agent on a specific spot or darkened skin area.

> **Cautions:** Be sure that any product you use contains no more than 2 percent hydroquinone, as higher concentrations can burn the skin. Up to 4 percent is available, but this should only be used under the guidance of a physician. Also, always apply a small amount to a test area to be sure you don't have an allergic or irritated reaction. Be careful to keep it away from your eyes and mucus membranes, far enough away that none will get in your eyes. If some does, wash it away with water; if irritation persists, which is rare, call your doctor.

Hydroquinone should only be used in conjunction with a stringent sun-protection program. It is best applied at night; but if you use it during the day, wear it *under* a good sunscreen. It will make you more sun-sensitive and sun exposure will negate some of the benefits. Remember that a tanning bed is just as bad for your skin as the sun.

Suggested brands. Palmer's Skin Success Eventone Fade Milk.

product	what it does	how it compares to RX products	cautions	some effective brands
Alpha-hydroxy/ Glycolic acid	Smoothes top layers of skin; evens skin tone	Not as effective	Can increase sun sensitivity; can sting sensitive individuals	M.D., Forté, SkinCeuticals Primacy line
Retinol	Increases growth of top layers of skin; some collagen stimulation	Not as effective	Can increase sun sensitivity; can sting sensitive individuals	Avon Anew, Affirm (Tx Systems), RoC
Furfurylade-nine	Improves skin texture; reduces fine wringkles; moisturizes	NA	No side effects	Kinerase, Kinetin
Copper peptides	Heals wounds; increases skin repair; stimulates formation of collagen	Very effective	No known side effects	Night therapy, Blue Copper Serum (Anagen.net), CP Serum (Skin Biology), Neova (ProCyte), Protect & Restore (Neutrogena)
Vitamin C creams	Antioxidant agent; helps stimulate collagen formation	Not as effective	Must be very acidic (pH=2.5) for best results	Any products in the Cellex-C line

Tri-Luma Cream: New Hope for the Mask of Melasma

As the name implies, this product is a combination of three ingredients: fluocinolone acetinide 0.01 percent (a topical steroid), hydroquinone 4 percent (the highest concentration of the bleaching cream), and tretinoin 0.05 percent (similar to vitamin A as discussed previously). This is the first triple-action cream for the treatment of moderate to severe melasma. It is more effective and seems to have fewer side effects than using the individual component products alone or in combination. Typical price is 30 grams for $95.

chapter eleven

cosmetics and makeup

Although we are firm believers in natural beauty, sometimes everyone needs a little bit of help from a jar or tube. For the most part, makeup has not changed very much in the last fifty years. Most products are still made primarily from oils, water, and colorings. However, just as the over-the-counter products mentioned in the last chapter contain active ingredients that are truly active, some modern cosmetics also contain ingredients that do more than just cover up or color imperfections.

Among the new products to look for are those that contain sunscreens, vitamins, and other ingredients that can make a difference in the actual health of your skin. There is also a new category of makeup products that use optical effects to affect the way you look.

decoding the ingredients in beauty products

Whether you opt for some of the nonsurgical procedures and treatments we recommend in this book, or simply choose to age naturally, there is no ignoring the fact that older skin is more delicate and more sensitive to irritants than younger skin. When you're young, you can get away with slathering any old formula on your skin, but as you mature, it's better to take care and learn exactly what goes into your favorite beauty products. If a product promises to deliver a certain benefit, make sure that it contains enough of the touted active ingredient to actually deliver that benefit. Below are a number of the most common types of ingredients found in over-the-counter products, along with a list of the most common chemicals within each type.

ANTIOXIDANTS

Among the most common antioxidants in many cosmetic products such as foundations are retinols and vitamins C and E (see chapter 10). In many cases, though, the percentage of active ingredient is much too small to have any real effect on the skin. Other antioxidants may be added as preservatives for the product itself. Among these: EDTA, BHA, grape seed extract, green tea extract, L-ergothioneine, and resveratrol.

EMOLLIENTS

Emollients are the ingredients that make your skin feel soft to the touch. They do this by actually penetrating the outer layer of the epidermis and making it softer and more pliable. Two of the most commonly used emollients are lanolin, a natural product of sheep skin and petrolatum, an ingredient of petroleum jelly. Vitamin E derivatives (tocopheryls) are also excellent emollients. Emollients tend to be greasy, and are usually used in small amounts in cosmetics. Many people are allergic to lanolin; if you are one of them, what may seem to be a dry-skin problem could turn out to be an allergy—be sure to read the labels!

Besides those mentioned, common emollients include: algae or seaweed extract, isopropyl isostearate, isopropyl palmitate (can cause blackheads or acne), mineral oil, capric/caprylic triglyceraldehydes, cholesterol, dimethicone/cyclomethicone, and a variety of natural oils, including almond, coconut, jojoba, avocado, sesame, sunflower, and grapeseed.

126

HUMECTANTS

These are natural ingredients that attract outside moisture to your skin (as opposed to moisturizers, which both add moisture and protect against its loss). Among the most commonly used, and generally non-allergenic, humectants are allantoin, ceramide(s), collagen, DNA, elastin, glycerin (also glycerol), hyaluronic acid (also called cyclic acid), lecithin (also helps the product to go on smoothly), panthenol, phospholipids, propylene glycol, pyrrolidone carboxylic acid (NA-PCA), sorbitol (a sugar), and urea, a natural component of sweat.

LUBRICANTS

These substances make the skin feel smoother to the touch. Cetyl alcohol (a lubricant that helps other ingredients to mix, and is not drying) and glycerin are commonly used lubricants.

PRESERVATIVES

Just as with food, cosmetics require preservatives to keep them from spoiling due to the growth of bacteria or molds. Although few cosmetics come with an expiration date on the label, contamination can be a problem; discard any old cosmetics you've had around for more than a year. Common preservatives include: ascorbyl palmitate, citric acid, diazolidinyl urea, EDTA (can cause dermatitis), ethanol, imidazolidinyl urea, octyl salicylate, parabens (methyl paraben, propyl paraben, butyl paraben), sodium borate, sorbic acid, triclosan, and quaternium-8, -14, or -15.

SOLVENTS

These are water or some form of alcohol; they are used to dissolve ingredients so they may be blended together. Some common solvents include: distilled, deionized, or purified water; acetylated lanolin alcohol (non-allergenic, but can cause pimples and blackheads); alcohol SD-40, or SDA-40.

OTHER INGREDIENTS

These include alpha-hydroxy acids (glycolic acid, citric acid, lactic acid, and malic acid, helpful in exfoliating and used as humectants), cellulose, often used as a thickener, ceramides (natural oils that help to hold your skin together).

Types of ceramides include: glycosphinogolipids, sphingolipids, glycolipids, phospholipids, cholesterol, and glycosylceramides. Some more ingredients: hydroquinone, a skin lightener (can be no more than 2 percent in over-the-counter products); isopropyl alcohol (antibacterial); liposomes (tiny spheres that encapsulate active ingredients and drugs for delivery into the skin); sodium laurel sulfate, a surfectant (cleansing agent) used in soaps and cleansers (can be irritating to sensitive skin); xanthan gum (thickener); propylene glycol (used as a base to carry other ingredients); and carmine (a dye).

INGREDIENTS THAT MAY BE DANGEROUS

Although they are not often found in cosmetics made by reputable companies, beware of ingredients such as formaldehyde and coal tar colors, which are known carcinogens.

Ingredients to Watch Out For

The following list of ingredients includes substances that may have legitimate uses in cosmetics but may also be added in tiny amounts for hype purposes. Don't believe everything you see in advertisements, and when in doubt, buy a product that you know is effective, such as the many products we recommend in this book.

Collagen. The fibrous support structure for the skin. Despite what ads may claim, you can't replace lost collagen by applying it to your skin. However, as a topical ingredient it is a good humectant, meaning it promotes the retention of water.

DNA. The genetic material of all cells, used as a humectant in some cosmetics. Beware of hype that promises special properties for DNA. It is simply another humectant.

Vitamins. Vitamins A, B, C, and E are often added to cosmetic products for various reasons. Variants of vitamin A, tretinoin, and retinol can help rejuvenate the skin, but only in specific forms and concentrations. B vitamins are essential in the diet, but there is no evidence that they can help the skin when applied topically. Vitamins C and E both have potent rejuvenating effects and also help to protect against sun damage, by inactivating free radicals, but only when supplied in specific forms in specific concentrations (see chapters 3 and 10).

choosing makeup

Today's makeup basics are the same as they were in your grandmother's day: makeup base, powder, cheek color; eye makeup, including masacara, shadow, liner, and brow color; lip liner and lipstick. A number of these, especially makeup bases, increasingly contain active ingredients, such as alpha-hydroxy acids, vitamins, and sunscreens, that are said to enhance and protect your complexion at the same time. The truth is that most of these products contain too small a percentage of the active ingredient to make a real difference in your appearance. Although modern makeup may go on easier and is certainly longer-lasting than the products used a generation ago, for most makeup categories, there's not much real news.

However, makeup bases and cover-ups have seen genuine improvements. Today they may contain not only sunscreens (always look for sun protection of 15 SPF and above), but also complexion brighteners, special pigments, and light-scattering pigments and particles that optically hide fine lines and discolorations.

You can now buy cover-ups and bases designed to change skin tones: cover-ups with a greenish color can minimize reddish or pinkish cast to the skin, while violet colored cover-ups minimize a sallow or yellowish look. Brighteners generally contain pinkish pigments to add a rosy glow to the face (not recommended if your skin already has a pink tone).

Light-scattering technology makes use of light-reflective pigments and crystals, such as powdered mother-of-pearl (conchiolin powder), micronized topaz powder, and micronized rose quartz powder, that direct light away from wrinkles and dark areas. These products give a glittering shine to the skin—some brands more than others—that tends to fade the longer you wear the product.

beauty care for men? the pros and cons

It's true that men are still a minority when it comes to skin care, but a growing one. We have seen the number of men seeking to improve their appearance continue to grow as more men discover how easy and hassle-free the new techniques make it to look younger and better. Many spas now offer special services to men clients, including scalp massage and facials. Some cosmetics companies have begun marketing skin products to men, including products containing the active ingredients we've told you about in this book, such as alpha-hydroxy acids, retinol, and vitamin C.

How to Have Beautiful Eyebrows
by Denise Chaplin, makeup artist and brow specialist
at John Barrett at Bergdorf Goodman

The appearance of your eyebrows is crucial to your over-all look. They should be sculpted, well-defined, and clean-looking. Well-shaped eyebrows create a frame for your face. They add lift, and bring out your eyes. If you have thick or straggly eyebrows, they can detract from your eyes. Taking a little heaviness away will let others notice your eyes more.

For shaping the brows, I prefer tweezing over waxing. Waxing was invented for quick hair removal, and for the rest of the body it's fine. It's good on any area where no design or sculpting is involved. But you simply can't shape as well with waxing. Also, it can be risky around the delicate eye area—you have to be very careful where you put the wax. If you use Renova or Retin-A, you mustn't use wax at all, because the wax can pull the top layer of skin right off, leading to scarring.

Many people find their brows change as they age. It's genetically determined. For some of us, the brows grow heavier, and the hairs may become wiry or curly. Yet many people continue to groom their brows the way they did when they were younger. Much of my work is in correcting brows. Sometimes they are too short from long-term waxing. After repeated waxings, the hairs just won't grow back, and you're stuck with the shape.

In deciding on eyebrow color, remember that in nature, your eyebrows are about two shades darker than your natural hair color. If you lighten or highlight your hair, change your eyebrow color accordingly.

No matter what condition your brows are in, there is always potential for beauty. If you have scanty, pale brows, make sure you keep them very clean and even. For this sort of brow, I prefer powder to pencil. Get a good brush with a slanted, angled edge, and brush the color through. You can use powdered eyeshadow (taupe is good) or special eyebrow powder, available from some fine cosmetics companies.

Although many people maintain beautiful eyebrows on their own, professional eyebrow grooming can be a big help if you're not good at your own tweezing. I'd recommend a professional grooming at least twice a year or more often, depending on how well you maintain it and how dark and thick your eyebrows grow. Many people do well with professional grooming ever two to six weeks. We put the shape in for you, then you keep it in between appointments.

cosmetics and makeup

A few companies, such as Studio5ive Skin System, even offer cosmetics made specifically for men, which, according to the Studio5ive web site (See Appendix B), are "virtually undetectable in any light or at any distance while enhancing a masculine, youthful, and healthy appearance." These products have somewhat different goals than women's cosmetics, but are said to improve the appearance of the skin, conceal blemishes, tame the eyebrows, and even enhance the beard shadow.

After all, just because a man is a grandfather doesn't mean he wants to look like one. There's a more practical reason as well: looking your best makes good business sense. Men in the public eye—models, actors, TV personalities, as well as those with high-profile jobs, such as salesmen and managers—may find that *not* looking their best can actually harm their advancement prospects.

A number of research studies have been done on the connection between attractiveness and job promotions or pay. Daniel Hamermesh, an economist at the University of Texas at Austin and the author of several papers on the connection between beauty and job success, has found that in several countries, including the United States, there is a pay premium of up to 5 percent for being very attractive. Likewise, people perceived as having below-average looks make up to ten percent less money than their average-looking counterparts.

This correlation between higher pay and better looks holds true for both men and women, which may explain why so many men are discovering the advantages of cosmetic treatments and products.

One group of men who have embraced the use of a particular treatment (Botox) is trial lawyers. According to *The Wall Street Journal*, some top male attorneys receive Botox treatments prior to facing a jury, so they will appear more sympathetic and less angry.

Looking better is not just about earnings for men or women, of course. Looking your best can markedly impact other important areas of your life. For example, improving your appearance can also improve your self-esteem, and, if you're among the growing number of middle-aged divorced men, can help you feel more competitive in the "meet market."

Men's new emphasis on looking good is a natural outgrowth of the trend toward a healthier lifestyle, according to Dr. James J. Romano, a prominent plastic surgeon in San Francisco. "Men more and more appreciate how plastic surgery and skin care support their total well-being, and are buying and using skin care products at an incredibly growing rate," Dr. Romano asserted. "These days, men are doing more than just showering, shaving, and combing their hair; they're having facials, nail care, massages. And why not? They have as much right to feel good about themselves as women do."

Youthful Makeup Tips for Older People
by Vivienne Mackinder, internationally known hair stylist and teacher, and four-time recipient of the North American hairdressing award

I believe that true beauty means to age with grace. Unlike our grandmothers, today we do have choices. We can mature with ease, keeping a fresh look while retaining the natural element.

Makeup, like hair color, needs to soften as we age. The tricks and tips you learned when you were a teenager, or even in your thirties, are no longer appropriate for an aging face.

As you grow older, your makeup application needs to become lighter. When you look in the mirror, you should see your overall beauty, not the makeup. Stay away from hard lines around the eyes, or overuse of contrasting lip pencils.

Foundation or base should be *light* and close to your natural skin tone, so that you do not look as though you are wearing a mask. Work with neutral colors around the eyes; use a good quality brush to apply your eye shadow, so that you can easily blend it, creating a soft, smoldering look.

Avoid too much under-eye makeup, as this can emphasize lines and creases under the eyes. Too much under eye-cover will crack, and the eye will appear more tired and old. Keep the mascara light also, and use an eyelash curler to open the eyes. Stay as natural as possible. Especially as you get older, remember, less is more!

The two most important features on the face to sculpt are the lips and eyebrows. The brow is the frame for the eye, and if it is not shaped correctly, you can look tired or sad. The brow should have a natural arch, creating the illusion of lift. Consider having your brows shaped professionally, and then you can maintain the look.

Visit a beauty salon for a makeover from a professional. Or go to your local cosmetic counter for a consultation and make-up lesson.

chapter twelve

how to keep your great new look

While each of the treatments we detail, or a combination of them, can certainly improve your appearance at any age, cosmetic procedures alone cannot make up for years of neglect, nor can they keep you looking young without some effort on your part. To look your best at all ages, practice good health habits. Eat well, exercise, and above all:

- **Avoid smoking.** It compromises the blood supply to your face, producing premature wrinkling and a sallow complexion. (For tips on stopping, see p. 136.)
- **Watch your weight.** Or, more accurately and perhaps surprisingly, avoid extreme fluctuations in your weight. Constantly gaining and then losing weight has a devastating effect on your skin, and the older you become, the

worse the effects. By the time you are middle aged, losing a few pounds will produce wrinkled, lax skin on your face and elsewhere on your body. (For nutrition information, see chapter 18.)

• **Use sun protection!** No matter where you live or what season it is, always use at least a 30 SPF sunscreen when you go outside. Remember that sun damage is cumulative. Every little bit hurts. When you're going to be out during the prime "sun hours" of 10 to 3, wear long sleeves and a brimmed hat. The sooner in life you start, the better. 90 percent of all sun damage occurs before the age of 22. (For much more on sun protection, see pp. 137–140).

START NONSURGICAL REJUVENATION TREATMENTS AS YOUNG AS POSSIBLE

In addition to the above sensible suggestions for a healthy lifestyle, it may also be a good idea to begin noninvasive cosmetic interventions while you and your skin are still young.

For example, most of the lines and wrinkles we've talked about in this book are dynamic wrinkles, caused by muscle movement. These lines can, with time and aging, become permanent in the skin, even when the muscles are not consciously being used. Although you can plump them up with fillers, you'll need to renew the treatment, and the muscles will continue to work in the same area, creating more lines. Using Botox to relax the muscles also helps, but once the lines have become permanent they will often still show, even when you are wearing a neutral expression.

However, we and many other physicians believe it is possible that if you start early enough, those permanent changes in the skin will never occur, or if they do will be far less obvious. For your own best possible look over a lifetime, we urge you to practice early intervention. Don't wait until your wrinkle or line problem is hopeless—go for treatment when it first becomes noticeable and it may not get much worse for a very long time.

Bear in mind that there is no one right age for beginning to use rejuvenating products or treatments. Someone who has spent a great deal of time in the sun might need help at age twenty-six, while someone in her mid-thirties might not need to do anything for several more years if she protects herself from sun damage and skin aging (by wearing a sunscreen and other protection), exercises, eats a balanced healthy diet, and keeps trim.

Finally, even after you have begun receiving treatments or using recommended products, continue to practice all the good habits listed above, especially with regard to smoking, avoiding weight fluctuations, and getting good sun protection. In addition, from your young adulthood, use one or more prescription skin products that have been proven to prevent and heal superficial aging changes. Among those we recommend are the following:

- Renova (see page 28)
- Vitamin C serums (see page 119)
- Kinerase (see page 115)
- Alpha hydroxy and glycolic acid creams and lotions (see pages 31 and 109)
- Copper sulfite preparations (see page 116)

the stop-smoking solution to clear, unwrinkled skin

In spite of everything, do you still smoke? It's nothing to be ashamed of, but it's definitely something to be changed, especially if you care about your looks. And it's something you *can* change, no matter how much or little you smoke or how long you've smoked.

We're not even going to mention all the health impairments smoking causes. We're sure you know them all—from the Surgeon General's warnings printed on the sides of cigarette packs and in ads, to the sad tales of friends and relatives succumbing to tobacco-caused diseases.

But what you may not know—and won't find printed in tiny print in cigarette ads—is that next to sun exposure, smoking is the most damaging thing you can do to your skin. And it harms your skin in many ways. The free radicals in smoke cause damage to all skin structures. Chemicals in the smoke restrict your blood flow, reducing the ability of your skin to take in the oxygen and nutrients it needs from the blood. Smoking causes your skin to look dull, lifeless, and baggy. The act of smoking itself creates or deepens wrinkles around your lips and eyes.

As if all this weren't enough, smoking makes you less attractive as a person. Your body and clothes always smell like smoke. Your hands and teeth develop brown stains from nicotine. Smoking reduces your energy level and makes it difficult, if not impossible, to get the exercise you need for health and vitality.

No matter how many cosmetic procedures or products you try, as long as you continue to smoke you can't possibly look your best. And the more years you smoke, the less your best may become. But—and this is the good news—

giving up smoking now will almost immediately begin to improve your appearance, and will help any cosmetic procedures enhance your looks to the fullest.

We know that smoking isn't easy to give up. It is, after all, an addiction. But millions of people have stopped smoking, and you can too. Following are some of the tips that we know work. For further information on smoking cessation, check the links in Appendix B.

TIPS TO SUCCESSFULLY KICK THE SMOKING HABIT

Keep trying. The majority of smokers who have succeeded in quitting have tried more than once—sometimes many times—before they finally succeeded.

Find a substitute. After you stop smoking you will probably feel jittery and restless. Part of this is withdrawal from nicotine, and part of it comes from the loss of an accustomed activity. Find something else to do with your hands—take up knitting or whittling. Find something else to stick in your mouth. Many ex-smokers find that chewing gum or sucking on a toothpick or even a hard candy helps.

Join a support group. While many people are able to quit on their own, having someone to share the experience with is often helpful. Join Smokenders, or a local group sponsored by your church or community. Check out support on the Internet. An especially good resource is About.Com's Quit Smoking site (see Appendix B for link).

Try nicotine gum or the patch. Although using nicotine gum or a patch prolongs your dependence on the drug, these aids have proven extremely helpful for many successful ex-smokers. One advantage is that you can use them even months after your last cigarette when stress causes you to want to light up again.

Exercise! Exercise is one of the best proven stress-relievers, and can help you deal with the stress of quitting as well as other stressors in your life. Not only will exercise make you feel better, the longer you go without smoking, the better you'll be able to exercise. Especially valuable are aerobic exercises, such as aerobic dance, step aerobics, and jogging; and exercises that focus on concentration and relaxation, such as t'ai chi and yoga. Another great anti-smoking exercise is walking. Whenever you feel the urge to light up, go for a walk—around the block or around the yard—until the urge passes.

Remember that there is no one right way to stop smoking. Whatever works for you is what's best. Don't be afraid to experiment. If one method doesn't work, try another. Studies have shown that using a combination of methods is the best way to quit for good. If you find all of this too difficult, contact your doctor. Prescription medications like Wellbutrin (Zyban) have made quitting easier for many people.

It should go without saying, but if you don't smoke—don't start!

don't forget the sunscreen!

Most of us love the sun and love doing things in the sun. Unfortunately, the sun doesn't love our skin; most of the aging changes detailed in this book are caused or made worse by too much sun exposure. And there's no such thing as "just a little" sun—every solar exposure, from the time you are a baby, damages your skin. The damage is cumulative; even a quick, unprotected trip to the mailbox will add to the total amount of damage and premature aging.

The good news is that you needn't turn into a troglodyte in order to protect your skin. Common sense, new sunscreen formulations, and high-tech clothing can combine to keep your complexion beautiful while you hike, play tennis, or otherwise enjoy the great outdoors in safety.

Remember the four Sun Safety S's:

- **Sunscreen your skin every day.** Be sure to cover all exposed areas, including the tops of your ears and feet, if you wear sandals.
- **Stay out of the sun between 11:00 and 4:00 P.M.** This is when the sun's burning rays are strongest. When you need to be out—say, on a hike—be sure to wear long sleeves and pants and a wide-brimmed hat.
- **Say goodbye to sunbathing.** It wasn't so long ago that a tanned skin looked healthy. But now when we see a "good" tan, we envision the premature wrinkles and unsightly spots that will cover it sooner rather than later. Sunbathing—just lying in the sun—is like suicide for your skin, and its effects are worse the lighter your natural skin color.
  If you must have a darker look, investigate some of the new self-tanning

> ## Ultraviolet A and B
>
> The two types of sunlight that cause skin damage are known as Ultraviolet A and B (UVA and UVB). Ultraviolet light is not visible, but packs enough energy to be absorbed by the skin and cause sunburn and other undesirable changes that can lead to premature aging and skin cancer. It used to be thought that only UVB, which is primarily responsible for sunburn, was dangerous, but now it's known that both types of radiation cause damage.

preparations. Look for those that contain dihydroxyacetone (DHA), which interacts with the top layer of your skin to produce a darkening effect, and is the only active ingredient approved by the FDA for sunless tanning. Unlike the self-tanning preparations of even a few years ago, modern self-tanners won't leave you streaked and orange.

• **Skip tanning beds.** Getting a tan through the use of tanning beds can be even worse than sunbathing outdoors. These machines make use of the same UV rays that cause a natural tan—and also cause skin damage. Studies have shown that premature skin aging is caused by both UVB and UVA, especially in chronic, low-dose exposures such as you would receive in an indoor tanning bed. Although most modern tanning machines produce mainly UVA, they also produce UVB, and both are harmful.

TOPICAL PROTECTION

Sunscreens have come a long way since they first became widely available in the 1970s. You can now buy sunscreens with protection ranging from minimal to extreme, and sunscreen ingredients are present in many cosmetic products, from facial lotions to makeup base. In fact, the field has become so crowded that the main problem is deciding which product(s) to use and when.

The most important thing to remember about sunscreens, whenever and wherever you purchase them, is to use them religiously. Unless you live in a cave and never venture outside during the day, you should apply sunscreen to all exposed areas of skin every day, all year round. If you want more evidence that much of skin aging is due to sun-caused damage and smoking, some Buddhist monks *do* live in caves. They seldom venture out in the sun, they don't smoke, and they have baby skin into their fifties, sixties, and seventies.

Sunscreens. Sunscreens—oils or lotions that you apply to your skin—
are designed to protect your skin from the effects of the sun's harmful UV
rays, both UVA and UVB (see box on page 136).

The strength of a topical sunscreen is measured by its SPF (sun protection
factor), which refers to how long the sunscreen will prevent your skin from reddening in the sun, compared to how long it would take to redden without any
protection. Thus, an SPF of 15 would theoretically allow you to stay in the sun
fifteen times longer than you could safely do without the sunscreen. If you usually turn red after ten minutes outside, with an SPF 15 cream you wouldn't
turn red for 150 minutes, or two and a half hours.

The Skin Cancer Foundation, a nonprofit organization that provides information on all aspects of skin cancers, recommends using an SPF of at least 15,
which blocks 93 percent of all UVB rays. Apply the preparation liberally, at
least twenty minutes before going outside, and reapply every two hours and
after swimming.

There is a catch to the use of topical sunscreen, however, which is that the
SPF measures only resistance to UVB rays. There is at present no standard like
the SPF rating to indicate how well a sunscreen protects against UVA. Most
sunscreens do provide protection against some UVA rays, especially those
advertised as providing broad-spectrum protection.

Most sunscreens have a shelf life of between three and four years. If the preparation is exposed to extreme heat (as in a hiking pack), its effectiveness may be
compromised. To be safe, discard sunscreen that is no longer white and creamy.

Bear in mind that no sunscreen fully protects your skin from the sun's rays.
To do that, you must also wear protective clothing and sunglasses, and avoid
the direct sun between 11:00 A.M. and 4:00 P.M.

Look for the following ingredients in your sunscreen. Protects against UVB:

- Octyl methoxycinnamate (can cause contact dermatitis)
- Octylmethyl cinnamate (OMC)
- PABA (para-aminobenzoic acid, seldom used because of potential for der-
  matitis)
- Padimate O
- Salicylates

Protects against UVA:

- Oxybenzone
- Avobenzone.

Sunblocks. Sunscreens provide a chemical barrier to the sun; their active ingredients absorb the sun's rays before they can damage your sin. Sunblocks, on the other hand, provide a physical barrier and are thus able to protect your skin more fully. You are probably familiar with sunblocks as that white paste (now pastel colors as well) you see on the nose and ears of many lifeguards. These preparations provide excellent broad spectrum protection, but most of us would not want to wear them when walking down the street or going to work.

The good news is that sunblocks have now entered the age of cosmetic elegance. The barrier incredients, titanium oxide and zinc oxide, are now microencapsulated, which means that they are chalky white at first, but as you smooth them on the skin they vanish. Voilá, protection without paste.

These products are especially valuable for those who have very sensitive skin, or who must be out in the sun a great deal (like lifeguards), and they are also valuable for the rest of us. Because they are usually more expensive than chemical sunscreens, sunblocks are more suitable for using on limited areas, such as the face, neck, ears, and backs of the hands.

Many companies make excellent sun blocks. Choose on the basis of active ingredients, feel, convenience, and cost. Sunscreens by Skinceuticals work very well, as do the Institute Beauté sunblocks available at our web site.

Antioxidant creams. Although these creams do not block the rays of the sun, evidence shows that antioxidants applied topically can help minimize sun damage by stimulating a skin-repairing enzyme (superoxide dismutase), and by helping to neutralize free radicals. Among the antioxidants we recommend are special cream formulations containing any or all of the following ingredients: vitamin C, vitamin E, copper, and co-enzyme Q10. Also good are products formulated from green tea extract (For more on vitamins C and E, see chapter 10.)

In addition to its other healthful benefits, vitamin C cream has been shown to (probably) help prevent the sun damage that leads to skin cancer when applied within 15 to 30 minutes of prolonged sun exposure. Likewise, natural vitamin E, in the form of d-alpha tocopherol, has also been shown to prevent UV damage. When combined in a sun-protective lotion, the vitamins can, between them, provide a formidable defense against the harmful changes caused by UV.

You might, in addition, want to consider supplementing your diet with extra vitamin C and vitamin E. A dose of 400 milligrams per day of vitamin E has been noted to reduce photodamage and wrinkles, and improve skin texture. It is believed that 500 to 1000 mg daily of vitamin C from food and/or supplements is also protective.

physical protection

Keeping the shirt on your back. In Victorian times, ladies never went anywhere outdoors without a parasol to protect their skin from the ravages of the sun. Today, we're all too active to restrict ourselves that way, but the idea of a physical barrier between your skin and the sun is as sound now as it was in great-great-grandma's day.

Experienced hikers and desert-dwellers know not to spend much time in the sun without long sleeves and trousers. But not all clothing is equally effective as a sun barrier. Especially in the summer, when the sun's rays are strongest and we tend to wear lightweight fabrics, those UV rays can easily penetrate even long sleeves, damaging the skin beneath. For example, a typical cotton t-shirt can allow up to 50 percent of UV rays to reach your skin (this is similar to an SPF of only 2). Get that T-shirt wet, as many do when wearing it as a protective cover-up in a swimming pool, and an additional 10 to 20 percent of the rays come through.

Fabrics that protect against the sun. So what can you do to protect yourself? No one wants to wear sticky sunscreen underneath clothing. Luckily, there's now another option: a growing number of manufacturers are making clothes out of new fabrics that have either been treated with sunscreen or have had sun screening fibers woven right in. These fabrics are made into a wide variety of clothing types and styles, including very lightweight cooling garments for the summer heat.
To evaluate sun-protective clothing, make sure the following questions are answered on the garment's label:

- Can the sun protection on the garment stand up to repeated washings?
- Does the garment provide at least a 30 SPF level of protection?
- Does the garment continue to protect even when wet (as from perspiration)?
- Is it safe for sensitive skin?

Among the fabrics most often used for sun-protective garb are Solarweave and Supplex.

Sun protection is more than a day at the beach. Though we're all primed to wear sun protection in the summer, be aware that the sun's rays are dangerous year round, and more dangerous the closer you get to the equator. The rays are also stronger the higher you go. Up on a mountaintop, it may feel cool, but the sun can be fierce and you should protect yourself from it. Be particularly cautious when skiing, as the snow can reflect the rays, adding to the direct sunlight on your skin. If you ski, you are probably very familiar with the red nose and face (except where protected by your ski goggles) that result from the sun exposure.

SEALS OF APPROVAL

The Skin Cancer Foundation evaluates sunscreens and sun-protective clothing. To be sure the product you have chosen is safe and effective, look for The Skin Cancer Foundation's Seal of Recommendation on the label. For more information on evaluation methods as well as other information on sun care products, visit the Skin Cancer Foundation website, listed in Appendix B.

The American Sun Protection Association, a nonprofit group representing manufacturers of sun-protection products, also offers a seal of approval to topical products and clothing that meet their standards for excellent sun protection. Look for their seal on products, or check their web site, listed in Appendix B.

preventing further age changes

Perhaps you've taken good care of yourself, utilized some of the procedures and products we recommend in this book, and reached middle age looking and feeling good, even though you no longer look twenty-two.

But how can you keep time's relentless march at bay for the next thirty or forty years? Is there anything you can do to maintain your present level of well-being and good looks?

The fortunate answer is yes—there is a lot you can do. You can follow the advice for younger readers given earlier in this chapter, and avail yourself of rejuvenating procedures early—before the changes become very visible and more difficult to treat. This also applies to renewal of procedures that you may have had recently, such as Botox to relax wrinkles or CoolTouch to rebuild collagen.

One of the most important things you can do to retain your youthful looks is to follow our suggestions for a healthy lifestyle, now and throughout your life. Most important, be aware of your body and its needs and take advantage of the wonderful new rejuvenating products.

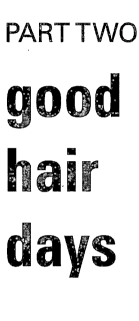

PART TWO

good hair days

how to have gorgeous hair at any age

A s we age, the problem is always either too little hair or too much and in the wrong place. In the next few pages, we'll take a look at the hows and whys of healthy, lustrous hair at all ages, as well as cutting-edge solutions for regrowing or replacing missing hair and removing unwanted hair.

how and why your hair changes with age

Some psychologists say that both men and women are more concerned about their hair than any other feature of their appearance. When you're young, your hair usually looks good no matter how you treat it. It mostly stays where it should be—on your head. It grows fast and looks healthy.

But as we get older—for some people sooner rather than later —the hair on the head becomes dry, flyaway, and breaks off, or worse, thins out. The hair on the body begins to sprout, very often in places where we'd much rather not have it. What causes all these hairy problems? Not surprisingly, the main causes of many of our bad hair days, or years, are the same suspects that wreak havoc with our skin: heat, sun, wind, water, environmental pollution (including ambient smoke), and just aging.

what is hair, exactly?

To see why these elements should affect the appearance of your hair, let's take a closer look at your crowning glory. Like your skin, the part of your hair that shows is made of dead, scaly protein tissue called keratin. An individual hair shaft is a kind of tube, with two main layers. The outer enclosing layer, is called the cuticle. It's made up of overlapping scales, like the shingles on a roof. The inner part of the hair shaft is filled with closely packed individual hair fibers, which determine your hair's strength, texture, and color. (There is a third innermost layer called the medulla, but it is only present in thick hairs, and it isn't generally affected by the elements or by hair-care products.)

The cuticle serves the same function for the inner part of your hair as the epidermis does for the inner part of your skin: it protects it from the onslaughts of the outside world. It's also the part of the hair that determines if your hair is shiny or dull, manageable or fly away. As long as nothing happens to harm the cuticle, it will remain intact and protective for about a year, and then it starts to wear away.

However, if the cuticle becomes damaged, the entire hair shaft is at risk. For example, when the cuticle wears down at the end of the shaft, the individual hair fibers begin to poke through, revealing the frazzled look of "split ends." There is no way to permanently repair damaged cuticle, so get a haircut. The best cure for split ends is to cut them off (though we will recommend some stop-gap measures to help damaged hair look good).

To compound the problem, your hair ages the same way your skin does—by producing fewer cells and producing them more slowly. Not only does the amount of hair you possess thin as you age, the hairs themselves tend to become thinner and weaker. Thus any damage you incur will seem more severe because it will be visible longer and appear more obvious.

Since the hair's cuticle is very easily damaged—more so the older you get—

one way to keep your hair looking healthy (and to keep your hair, period) is to minimize exposure to all the things that can harm it, which include not only hair coloring, curling, and straightening, but also blow-drying, UV rays, chlorine, salt water, heat, and products containing alcohol. If this sounds to you like a recipe for a completely inactive life, you are right. The fact is that today's active lifestyles are *not* good for our hair, but inactive lifestyles are bad for our bodies and souls. What to do? Luckily, there are a number of new products and treatments that are actually good for the hair, and we'll examine them later on in this chapter.

How the Right Haircut Can Make You Look Younger and Other Tricks of the Trade

by Vivian Mackinder, internationally known hairstylist and teacher, and four-time recipient of the North American Hairdressing Award

Defying one's age is as old as time itself. As a hairstylist based in a top New York salon, my challenge is to create an image for my clients that is fashionable, helps them feel comfortable in their own skin, enhances their lifestyle, and develops their full beauty potential, whatever their age.

"The only constant in life is change" —Confucius. I've always liked this saying, because to me it reflects a truth about beauty and the nature of change. Whenever you dramatically change one aspect of your appearance, it always impacts another area. It's like painting only the trim of your house. If you did that, the trim would look great, but the rest of the house would then appear shabby. Remodeling your hair or your face is the same thing. For example, if you've had your skin rejuvenated by some of the great techniques discussed in this book, you'll look even better if you get your makeup and hair updated too.

This is one reason I recommend investing the time and money to have your look created by a professional, who has the experience and objectivity to consider not only the details but the big picture. When you look good, you feel good, and your positive energy attracts good opportunities into your life. The following hairstyling tips are mainly for women, but men can learn a thing or two from them as well.

The Advantages of a Terrific Haircut

- **Hair and the face.** Part of what makes young people look young is their bone structure. Their cheekbones and jaw lines are firm and prominent, giving a lift to the face. Sadly, as we age, the facial muscles and skin tone migrate south, obscuring that clean bone structure. For a youthful look we must create the illusion of lift, drawing the hair internally or externally away from the face.

- **Facial shape.** The classic, youthful face shape is considered to be oval. Choose a hair-style designed to create the illusion of an oval face.
- **Length.** Long hair is associated with children and teens. Believe me when I tell you that long hair becomes harder to wear as we age, and I don't just mean that it's harder to handle. Long, hanging hair drags the features down.
- **A good haircut can take ten years off your appearance.** Would you wear your old prom dress? Of course not. So why would you wear the same hairstyle you wore then? An old hairstyle gives the impression of being stuck in a time warp.
- **Classical beauty.** In our teens we could be trendy, breaking the rules and having fun with fashion and hairstyles. After all, youth was on our side. As we mature, we need to be a bit more conservative. We need to translate and interpret the current trends into softer, classic forms to go with the softening of our features.
- **A great haircut makes your hair itself look more youthful.** For example, a blunt cut is the best type of trim for minimizing split ends, reflecting shine, and having a healthy bounce (a razor cut, which cuts the hair on a slant rather than straight across, simply exposes more of the hair fibers inside the cuticle to the outside). Choose a fashionable current style that is classic rather than trendy, like a "bob." The trick is to think style and shape, not inches. It's time to trade those long tresses in for a style that fits your bone structure and enhances your beauty.

Choosing the Perfect Hairstyle

- **What sorts of lines are best?** I believe that for mature women, hair shapes need to be soft, feminine, and classic, with a fashion twist if it's appropriate for your hair and face type. Hard lines within a style can make you look harsh, because the lines of the haircut emphasize the lines on the face. Remember that fashion is fleeting, but style is timeless.
- **What is your lifestyle?** If you're very athletic, for example, constantly playing tennis or jogging, you'll need a different hairdo than someone who spends more time in sedentary pursuits.
- **What is your overall image that you want to present?** Are you classic, country, sporty, corporate, cute, androgynous, glamorous, or sexy? Be sure that your beauty image fits your total image and lifestyle.

- **Are you fashion savvy or conservative?** Your choice of a suitable hairdo depends on how you dress.
- **What's your body type?** A hairstyle has to work with balance and proportion, meaning how the scale of the style relates to both body type and fashion silhouette. If you have a very large head, you'll need a do that is proportional; the same is true for a very small head.
- **What's your face shape?** What's your best feature? What do you want to emphasize or distract the eye away from?
- **What is your hair's texture?** If you have thin, fine hair, there is no way you can have an elaborate hairstyle that requires lots of body and bounce.
- **What is your skin tone?** Does it work with your current hair color? If not, what color would be better? Is your overall look cool or warm? Hair color can be a big trauma for some people. Try a "salon color consultation kit" that contains head bands with different-colored bangs you can use as a color preview. Believe me, it's hard to evaluate the effect of a hair color selection by looking at a color chart. If your professional salon doesn't offer color consultation kits, go to a wig store and try on wigs in various colors.
- **How much time and money do you have to put into hair maintenance?** Don't underestimate the impact a new hairstyle can make on your life, one aspect being time. If you aren't willing to spend much time on the upkeep, you're better off with a simple style that requires minimal processing.

space-age products that make your hair look great

Once you've found the perfect hairdo and color, your aim is to keep your hair thick, shiny, and glossy (or make it appear that way). Modern technology has created products that can work wonders with even thin, fine hair. Here's what to look for in hair products:

SHAMPOOS

To keep your hair looking its best, you need to use specially formulated shampoos. Modern shampoos use cleansers called surfactants, which clean well and rinse out completely. Two of the most common surfactants are ammonium lauryl sulphate and ammonium laureth sulphate.

Most shampoos also include conditioning ingredients, usually silicones, to keep hair smooth and shiny. Other ingredients may include thickening agents, colorings, and preservatives. Shampoos formulated for oily hair will contain less of conditioning ingredients, while dry-hair shampoos will contain more. Shampoos meant to treat dandruff contain zinc pyrithione.

Most brand-name shampoos, either those purchased in a drugstore or a salon, will work well. What's important is to choose a shampoo made for your type of hair.

> **Note:** For fine, thin hair, the Nioxin brand, available in beauty salons and on the Internet, is especially good (see Appendix B for link).

CONDITIONERS

Today's understanding of hair structure coupled with science and technology have produced conditioners that go beyond the superficial; they make your hair look good while actually nourishing it.

While conditioners cannot repair damage, they can increase shine, decrease static electricity, improve hair strength, and provide ultraviolet (UV) radiation protection.

Ingredients to look for:

- For shine. Look for products with polymer film-forming agents, such as methacrylate derivatives, which increase hair shine by helping the cuticle scales to lie flat against the hair shaft.
- For flyaway hair. Combing or brushing your hair creates static electricity. The individual hair shafts become negatively charged and repel each other, preventing the hair from lying smoothly. Conditioners that contain quaternary ammonium minimize static electricity by giving a positive charge to the hair and helping to neutralize the static.

> **Note:** in an emergency you can tame flyaways by gently rubbing an anti-static dryer sheet over your hair.

- For weak, damaged hair, including hair that has been overprocessed, look for hydrolyzed proteins or hydrolized human hair keratin proteins to increase the hair's strength. These ingredients are small molecules that can penetrate the cuticle to nourish the inner core of the hair. Dimethicone can help prevent further damage by making your hair less resistant to combing and brushing. Collagen, silk protein, and panthenol (vitamin B5) can also help weak hair by penetrating the hair shaft and increasing its moisture content.
- For split ends. Although damaged hair cuticles cannot be repaired, some conditioners are able to glue the ends together so effectively that they appear to vanish even under a magnifying glass. Look for dimethicone, a silicone compound. Unfortunately, the "glue" effect is only temporary, so the next time you wash your hair, the splits will reappear. Hydrolyzed proteins and hydrolized human hair keratin proteins are also helpful in disguising split ends.
- Sunburned hair. Although hair can't develop cancer, the sun damages it as surely as it damages your skin. Ultraviolet exposure causes oxidation of molecules within the hair shaft that are important for hair strength. If this oxidation occurs, the hair becomes weak, dry, rough, faded, and brittle. The sun is also hard on lightened hair: blond hair may develop "photo-yellowing," in which the sun's rays cause yellowing, fading, and a dull appearance. Darker hair can also change color, as the sun causes the natural melanin in the hair shaft to fade and appear reddish.

  To sun-proof your hair, look for a leave-in conditioner that contains zinc oxide. Always wear a hat made of a solid material that covers your whole head. Straw hats may look great, but they don't do a good job of protecting your hair from the sun.
- Fine, thin hair. Don't resist using conditioners if you have fine hair because the conditioner can make you think it looks even thinner. Instead, look for a conditioner made especially for fine, thin hair, and use it sparingly and only on the ends.

VOLUMIZERS

Volumizers can make thin or fine hair appear thicker and full of body. They are usually applied after washing and before styling (though some shampoos contain volumizers). There are two main types of volumizers: the more traditional ones add thickness by depositing chemicals on the outside of the hair shaft. A number of new products actually penetrate the cuticle, causing the hair itself to expand. Although the measurable increase in diameter of the hair is small, every little bit helps, especially when you're dealing with literally thousands of hairs.

You may need to experiment to see which sort of volumizer works best with your hair. Ingredients in the type that coats the hair shaft are mostly liquid resins. Ingredients that work from within the hair shaft include keratin and collagen, which can increase the moisture within the shaft and thus swell it.

For fine, thin, limp hair, root lifters are designed to coat the root of the hair shaft, lifting it away from the head and adding body. Look for resins and algae.

damage control

All experts insist that you can't truly repair hair once it has been damaged, but using conditioners with the ingredients listed above can go a long way to improving your hair's appearance. Also recommended are periodic deep-conditioning treatments, which can actually penetrate the hair shaft; and getting your frazzled ends trimmed regularly will help you to preserve your crowning glory.

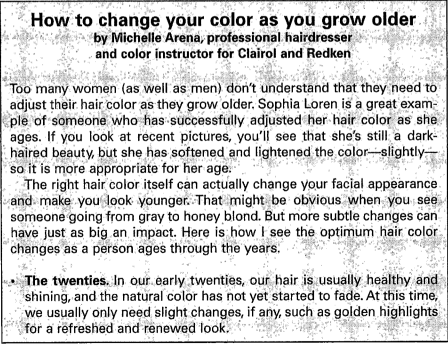

How to change your color as you grow older
by Michelle Arena, professional hairdresser
and color instructor for Clairol and Redken

Too many women (as well as men) don't understand that they need to adjust their hair color as they grow older. Sophia Loren is a great example of someone who has successfully adjusted her hair color as she ages. If you look at recent pictures, you'll see that she's still a dark-haired beauty, but she has softened and lightened the color—slightly—so it is more appropriate for her age.

The right hair color itself can actually change your facial appearance and make you look younger. That might be obvious when you see someone going from gray to honey blond. But more subtle changes can have just as big an impact. Here is how I see the optimum hair color changes as a person ages through the years.

- **The twenties.** In our early twenties, our hair is usually healthy and shining, and the natural color has not yet started to fade. At this time, we usually only need slight changes, if any, such as golden highlights for a refreshed and renewed look.

- **The thirties.** In this decade, our hair still has most of its original color, but strands of gray may be starting to show. We're usually busy with family and career, and need to look our best with not much time to do it in. This is a great time to add more highlights, or else blend our gray hair with semi-permanent hair colors that don't change the natural color.
- **The forties (and often starting in the late thirties).** The stresses of family, job, and life combine with beginnings of hormonal changes to cause the hair to lose its natural vitality, color, and shine. The gray hairs may be too numerous to cover up at this point, so it's time to go to permanent hair color to not only cover the gray, but—and this is important—to lighten and soften your natural color so it is more appropriate for your older skin.
- **The fifties to mid-sixties.** After our children are grown and we're beginning to spoil our grandchildren, it's definitely time to go noticeably lighter, unless the hair is already light, in which case you need to soften the color by adding highlights to permanent hair color.
- **The seventies and beyond.** This is when it's a good idea to continue to evaluate the balance of the skin's color and the hair color. Now is when you may choose to let your hair go gray or white or continue to wear a toned-down version of the color you were born with or have worn for several decades. That's the great thing about living in the twenty-first century. No one look is required, and many options exist for continued beauty, even into old age.

Color Tips for the Over-Thirties

- Dark solid colors (brown or black) can be very aging. Wearing these dark colors is the surest way to accentuate every facial line and wrinkle. Remember that as we age both our skin tone and hair color lose pigment. That's why it's best to stay with soft colors.
- If you're blonde, be careful not to go too light or brassy; both of these can look hard and unsophisticated. Remember that you want some contrast between your hair and skin colors.
- Don't overdo the highlights. Highlights are fine, but know when to stop before your skin and hair are the same color. This never looks good. Remember that more is not always better!

chapter fourteen

too
little
hair

H air tends to grow sparser with age. That's simply one of the facts of life. Unfortunately, thin or balding hair can be aging. This is a problem for both men and women, but even more so for men, and since it can even begin in the early twenties. It's no wonder that so many men (and women) try virtually anything to slow or stop their hair from thinning. (Though not everyone is unhappy with baldness. See the box on page 160 for another view.)

You probably already know that for most men, pattern baldness is inherited. For many men, the pattern of hair loss is in the familiar horseshoe shape, where a fringe of hair is left around the sides and back. Other men lose hair primarily from the crown, or their hair recedes at the forehead line. Contrary to popular opinion, the genes for hair loss can be passed down on either side of the family. If your father was bald, you're very likely to be bald too, and in the same pattern.

baldness does not discriminate

What you may not know is that many women inherit the same genes. They suffer through the thinning of the hair (though usually not complete baldness) in exactly the same areas of the scalp, usually the crown and forehead. This doesn't usually begin until menopause, when the natural male hormones that are always present become relatively stronger as estrogen decreases.

Although hair loss is usually gradual, it may seem to come about all at once. About 90 percent of the hair on a person's scalp is growing at any one time, and for each given hair this growth phase lasts between two and six years. The remaining ten percent of the hair is in a resting phase that lasts two to three months, at the end of which it falls out. Ordinarily, a new hair will then begin to grow from the same follicle, but once pattern baldness sets in, the follicle may begin to shrink and eventually shut down.

other causes of baldness

In addition to male pattern baldness, there are many other, though less likely, causes of thinning hair. Alopecia, as hair loss is called technically, can be caused by a number of illnesses, including thyroid disease, malnutrition, hormonal fluctuations (most common in women during pregnancy and menopause), or allergies. It can also be caused by over-processing or too-vigorous styling, or by chemotherapy and some other medications (but in these cases the hair will almost always grow back.) In some cases, the cause of hair loss may remain unknown even after a thorough medical investigation. Nevertheless, it's important to get a medical evaluation if your hair suddenly begins falling out, as it could be a symptom of a medical problem that needs immediate treatment.

Where to get help

It's usually best to visit a dermatologist, who will ask about your general health and medical background, including all medications and supplements you take, your family history of hair loss, and any recent illnesses.

Many of the causes of thinning hair and baldness do have cures, which usually involve simply letting the hair grow back out, which it will usually do. This is particularly effective in cases where the hair was damaged by over-processing.

In cases involving male pattern baldness, however, until recent times there was little that could be done. Today, though there is still no cure for pattern baldness, there are many solutions, and the number of possibilities is growing.

New drugs can actually halt hair loss and to some extent cause hair to regrow. New medical technologies can provide semi-permanent and temporary hair replacements. If you choose to get a wig or toupee, the choices today are better and more natural looking than ever.

The following treatments and strategies are the space-age answer to the age-old problem of genetic hair loss. Unless otherwise noted, they work equally well for women and men.

DRUGS

Minoxidil and generics. Originally formulated as a treatment for high blood-pressure, minoxidil, first marketed under the trade name Rogaine, is now available over-the-counter to treat male pattern baldness. It's not known exactly how minoxidil works to stimulate the hair follicles, and its effects vary depending from person to person. It generally works better on people whose hair loss has not progressed too far. Although it does result in some amount of regrowth of hair, minoxidil is best at preventing further hair loss.

To use minoxidil, rub it into your scalp twice a day, and leave it on for a minimum of four hours. There are generally no side effects except, rarely, contact dermatitis. Products containing 2 percent minoxidil work for both men and women, while 5 percent solutions should be used only by men (they can cause facial hair growth in women).

The 2 percent version will take effect within four months to a year, while a 5 percent product, which causes more and thicker hair growth, can be effective within four months. Prices range from $42.95 to nearly ninety dollars for a three-month supply (three bottles). Shop around and look for Internet specials.

The DHT Connection. DHT, a derivative of testosterone, is believed by some researchers to be the chemical that turns on the gene for male pattern baldness, causing the hair follicles to shrink and eventually stop working. Researchers say that while genetics are important in this sort of baldness, stress, diet, and a predisposition to the effects of DHT also play a role. Natural supplements and some foods are said to help block the effects of DHT, but none of these remedies has yet been scientifically proven. A number of promising new treatments for baldness work by turning DHT off or preventing its formation in the first place.

Finasteride. This drug, originally developed for use by men with enlarged prostates, under the name Proscar, blocks the formation of DHT in the hair follicle. It was noticed that balding men on the drug began to regrow hair, and a lower dosage of the drug was approved by the FDA under the trade name Propecia, as a treatment for male pattern baldness.

Finasteride may be the ultimate answer for many men, as it prevents the shrinking of hair follicles that leads to hair loss. It also permits modest regrowth of hair. There is evidence that when finasteride is combined with minoxidil, the amount and quality of new hair growth is greater than with either drug alone. Be sure to consult your doctor before combining these treatments.

Finasteride has few side effects, but *must never be used—or even touched—by pregnant or lactating women,* because it could affect male embryos or infants. Among the side effects possible (in men) are decreased volume of ejaculation, impotence, decreased sex drive, difficulty with urination, dizziness, headache, and weakness.

Finasteride can be taken either as a tablet or a lotion applied to the scalp. The cost of 30 tablets of finasteride ranges from $40 to $125. Be sure to compare prices before buying. By the way, the only difference between Proscar and Propecia is the dose (the amount of finasteride in each pill). Because Proscar is considerably less expensive, many users save money by buying Proscar and breaking the tablet into five pieces (Propecia comes in 1 mg tablets and Proscar in 5 mg tablets).

The value of finasteride in women has not been evaluated.

Aldactone. The brand name for spironolactone is a diuretic that does double-duty as a hair-restorer. Like finasteride, it interferes with the activity of DHT in the hair follicles. It is much more potent in its hair-restoring abilities than finasteride, but can cause serious side effects in men, ranging from impotence to breast enlargement. It appears to be effective in women without serious side effects, however.

Because this drug can have such serious side effects, you should only take it under a doctor's supervision. Never take it with any other diuretic, or with any medication that contains potassium. Aldactone is relatively inexpensive, costing around $30 to 35 for 100 pills.

Future treatments. A frenzy of research is discovering new drugs and treatments to prevent or cure baldness. Among the promising upcoming treatments are new drugs affecting DHT, such as Fluridil, which blocks the receptors for DHT in the hair follicle. A new, experimental, surgical technique involves culturing hair follicles from a still-productive part of the scalp, then injecting them into the barren areas to provide new growth. For up-to-the-minute news, check out Regrowth.com on the Web, which offers comprehensive coverage of all aspects of male pattern baldness (see Appendix B for link).

HAIR SOLUTIONS

Weaves, wigs, toupees, and hair extensions. Thanks to modern technology, there are literally thousands of types of hair prosthetics, using synthetics or natural hair, and ranging from full wigs to toupees or hair pieces, from removable to semi-permanently attached, and including "fun" hair extensions and weaves (mainly for women). Many relatively inexpensive wigs can serve as useful cover-ups for baldness resulting from chemotherapy, but for a long-term look for balding men, the best hair solution is to purchase a very good custom toupee or hairpiece and to be willing to invest in its upkeep.

Be aware that a custom-designed hair-piece is not cheap: they can cost up to $4,000, and, depending on the type of product, yearly maintenance can cost from $500 to more than $1,000. In our opinion, nothing looks worse than a poorly made or poorly fitted hairpiece, so, if this is the solution you choose, we recommend that you purchase the best hair piece that you can. If it doesn't look natural, it will make you look far older than a receding hairline.

No ponytails or comb-overs, please! Perhaps because they have been somewhat less concerned with their appearance throughout their lives than women have, aging men sometimes arrive at bizarre solutions to the loss of their locks (and youth). We've all known men of a certain age who suddenly dumped their wives of many years, bought a sports car, and grew a ponytail.

Please believe us when we tell you that a ponytail is *not* an attractive option for most men older than their early twenties. Even worse is the comb-over, in which a man lets his remaining fringe of hair grow long and then plasters it over the bald spot. Nothing can look worse, except perhaps a very bad toupee. On the other hand, an attractive man who happens to be bald is still an attractive man who doesn't have bad hair (fake or real) to detract from his appearance.

Surgical solutions. Because the focus of this book is on non-surgical solutions to problems of aging, we will briefly mention the surgical treatments for hair loss. The two most common procedures are hair transplants or implants and scalp reductions.

Transplants, which were first performed in the 1950s, involves transplanting small plugs of hair-containing scalp from areas where hair still grows to those where it doesn't. Early grafts were expensive and often produced cosmetically unnatural results. Since then, the technique has improved, and the right surgeon can often achieve very natural-looking results. However, it is extremely important to choose a surgeon who not only possesses extensive experience in hair transplantation, but who also has an aesthetic and artistic sense.

Scalp reductions, which are useful only to those men who have a bald spot in the crown area of their scalp, involves removing an elliptical section of the balding portion of the scalp and stretching the hair-bearing portion along the sides toward the middle.

Other procedures include the trademarked "Hairlift," which, like a scalp reduction, stretches the hair-bearing part of the scalp upward and forward, and, when combined with hair transplantation to the hairline, can produce very natural-looking hair, even on men with extensive baldness. For more information on the Hairlift and other procedures, see the web site for Dominic A. Brandy, M.D., listed in Appendix B.

An Appreciation of Bald Men

While to some people bald means "old," for others it's a definite turn-on. After all, baldness signals that a man's testosterone is working, and what could be sexier than that?

It's really true, some men find that they are now considered more attractive with less on top. Several top movie stars, including Bob Hoskins and Sean Connery, are known for their baldness—and their devastating effect on women. Another, much younger, but equally charismatic actor is Michael Rosenbaum, the young co-star of TV's *Smallville*. Though Rosenbaum still has his own hair in real life, he plays Lex Luthor with a shaved head, and is currently one of the leading heartthrobs for today's teens and young women.

Melba Newsome, a successful forty-something journalist, says she has always found bald men attractive. Newsome says, "When men go on and on about losing their hair I say, 'Michael Jordan. Yul Brynner. Sean Connery.'"

If you're currently partly bald and want to go all the way, see chapter 15.

chapter fifteen

how to get rid of unwanted hair

Too much hair, or hair in the wrong places, is one of the side-effects of aging that your mother probably never told you about. Men expect to grow facial hair, but women don't. Yet a surprisingly large number of women do grow hair on their faces—and they become hairier as they get older. Hair on the upper lips, hair on the cheeks, hair on the legs and arms and under the arms—even hair on the chest and hair on the breasts!

For men, hair is expected to grow in all those places, but it may also start sprouting in places where it may not be wanted, such as on the back, or on the ears (and even *from* the ears). Until fairly recently, there was little that could be done about any of these problems short of shaving, waxing, depilatories (all short-term treatments), and electrolysis (long-term, but extraordinarily tedious and time-consuming). Today we can offer a number of simple in-office, non-surgical procedures that will make those unwanted hairs a distant memory. Permanently.

There are a number of reasons in addition to aging that can cause excessive facial and body hair. Among them are heredity (those of Mediterranean descent, for example, tend to be hairier than Asians or those with Scandinavian ancestors) and certain medical conditions, including an excess of male hormone, reactions to certain drugs, and polycystic ovarian syndrome, a fairly rare condition in women that can also result in infertility. If you suspect your excessive hairiness may have a medical cause, be sure to speak to your primary care physician about it.

do-it yourself or at-home methods of hair removal

For most people with too much hair, however, the main causes are aging and genetics. Fortunately, there are a number of new procedures and products, as well as improvements on old ones, that make going hairless easier than ever.

Depilatories. Depilatories have been used for decades by women who don't want rough skin on their legs or face from shaving. These products, made of acids such as sodium thioglycolate or calcium thioglycolate, break down the protein structure of the hair. After the depilatory has been left on the skin for a given period of time (usually five to ten minutes), the hair dissolves (to just below the skin line) and can be rinsed off.

Depilatories are great for a fast, effective treatment, but because the chemicals used are harsh, they can easily cause skin irritation. Also, they are not a permanent solution, and need to be reapplied whenever new hair growth becomes obvious.

Depilatories should be applied in a smooth, thick layer, but not rubbed in. Depilatory manufacturers recommend applying a small, test amount of the product to the inside of the elbow before general use. If there is no reaction after twenty-four hours, it should be safe to use on a bigger area. It's important to follow the directions for the amount of time to leave the product on; exceeding the recommended time could result in burning or inflammation. Be sure to thoroughly rinse the skin after use.

Depilatories work best when applied after a warm bath or shower, when the hairs are softer and the pores are open. They tend to work better on light-colored and less coarse hair, and should not be used if there are open sores or irritated areas on the skin, or within a few days after a sunburn.

PRESCRIPTION HAIR REMOVAL

Vaniqua. Vaniqua is the brand name of Eflornithine Hcl, a prescription cream that has recently been approved by the FDA for facial hair removal in women. It works by blocking an enzyme that is necessary for hair growth, and has been clinically proven to decrease the growth of facial hair. Although Vaniqua doesn't work on all women (clinical trials showed it was effective in approximately two thirds of women who tried it), its results become apparent after only two months of use. Side effects are minimal, and include minor skin irritation, such as stinging, redness, and hair bumps.

Vaniqua needs to be used twice a day, eight hours apart. To use it, massage a very small amount of Vaniqua in a thin layer over the targeted area of skin. Apply it after cleansing your face and before applying cosmetics or sunscreen. Wait at least four hours after application before washing your face again. Until Vaniqua starts to work, you'll need to continue with your current method of hair removal.

Vaniqua makes daily shaving or tweezing a thing of the past, though you'll still need to attend to stray hairs every few days. Bear in mind that if you stop using Vaniqua, your hair will begin to regrow at its old rate. Another drawback to Vaniqua is that it is pricey: a 30-gram tube, which lasts several weeks, costs from a little over $100 to $150 on the Internet.

PROFESSIONAL METHODS OF HAIR REMOVAL

Waxing. Waxing, a hair-removal solution in which hot wax is applied to the skin and then removed (along with unwanted hair), is a fairly long-lasting procedure that is most often used on eyebrows, the moustache area, legs, and the bikini line. This is not always a good method if you have dark skin, as it may cause pigment changes.

Professional waxing varies in cost depending on the part of the body to be waxed. Typical costs range from about $15 for eyebrow or upper lip waxing to around $50 for full leg and bikini wax for women or full back wax for men.

Results generally last four to six weeks, depending on how fast your hair grows and how dark it is.

Electrolysis. Until recently, electrolysis was the only permanent method of hair removal. In electrolysis, a trained and skilled operator removes hairs individually by inserting a tiny needle into each hair follicle and zapping it with electricity, which kills the hair follicle. The hair within the follicle is then removed with a tweezers.

Complete electrolysis of a given skin area can take many treatments because not all hair follicles respond to a first treatment, and any follicles that are in the resting stage during treatment can't be treated until they become active again. Electroysis sessions are typically only fifteen minutes long—because that is about the maximum that most people can take. One or two sessions per week is also typical, with the upper lip taking a year or more to complete. Larger areas, such as legs or the back, are truly daunting tasks. If done improperly, electrolysis can cause deeply pitted scarring. Even when done properly, electrolysis can cause skin pigment changes, especially in people of color.

Electrolysis works best on women with white or light-colored hair; in fact, for white or light-gray hair, electrolysis is currently the only option for long-term hair removal, because current lasers work poorly or not at all on white or light-gray hair.

Electrolysis is not cheap, ranging from $25 to $150 an hour. Bear in mind that the cost will be spread out over several weeks, months, or years, depending on the extent of the area from which you wish to remove hair.

Although do-it-yourself electrolysis kits are available, this procedure can potentially damage or scar your skin, so it should only be performed by a trained professional. To find a board-certified electrologist in your area, check the American Electrology Association (see web link in Appendix B).

LASER HAIR REMOVAL— "THE FINAL ANSWER?"

Annette, a thirty-six-year-old media buyer, is a Mediterranean beauty with a secret. "I have hair on my face. Dark, thick, hair. I have to shave my face every morning. I don't leave the house until I do," she admitted.

For years, Annette tried waxing, plucking, and electrolysis. "Nothing worked," she sighed. "For good results from electrolysis, I would have had to spend more time with the electrologist than with my boyfriend."

Luckily for her, Annette heard about laser removal of unwanted hair. "I wouldn't exactly call it fun," she reported. "In fact, it hurts! But it hurts less than electrolysis. I had my first session two months ago, and since then I've had two more sessions, to my chin, upper lip, and sideburn areas. Each procedure lasted about twenty minutes. By the time I left the office, the soreness and redness were almost gone. I still shave my face, but now only once or twice a week, and with a few more sessions, I won't have to shave ever again."

Laser hair removal may indeed be the final answer to unwanted hair. Hair-removal lasers work by selectively targeting the melanin pigment in your hair follicle, which destroys the hair follicle and prevents future hair growth. The lighter your hair, the more treatments you will need (because there is less melanin for the laser to home in on). Current laser hair removal doesn't work on white hair, and is only slightly effective on very light blond or very light gray hair and fine vellus hair (fine, non-pigmented body hair).

Laser hair removal is far superior to all other methods. Unlike electrolysis and waxing, it is relatively painless, and because it targets more than one follicle at a time (a hundred or more), it can be used on larger areas of skin like the back and chest. If you so desire, you can go bare from nose to toes. (We do not recommend using lasers for the eye area below the eyebrows because of the remote possibility of eye damage.) Laser hair removal has minimal side effects, and these are usually no more than slight redness or irritation that quickly goes away.

Laser hair removal only works when a hair is in the follicle. Not all of your follicles will simultaneously be in the optimum, growing stage during a laser session, so you will require several treatments. Depending on the area to be treated, and the relative hairiness of the area, count on at least three to six treatments, approximately six weeks apart. If you are having your face treated, you will probably need periodic touch-ups for several months until all the follicles have been destroyed.

Laser hair removal is about one to two thousand times faster than electrolysis. If a good electrologist can remove six hairs a minute, she will remove fewer than one hundred hairs in a typical fifteen-minute session. A hair removal laser can treat as many as one hundred hairs or more with each pulse, and commonly pulses once or twice per second. Your back probably has a few hundred thousand hair follicles. A laser hair removal treatment of your back will take about one hour. Electrolysis at one hundred hairs per fifteen minutes will take years.

We use two different lasers for hair removal:

The Apogee laser. A long-pulse Alexandrite laser made by Cynosure, and used for people with light- or medium-color skin. Similar lasers include the Candela GentleLASE. Caution should be used if there is a suntan or sunburn, and in that case we usually postpone treatment for a few weeks. These lasers work well for dark, light, and finer hair.

The Lyra laser. This long-pulse Nd:YAG-erbium laser from Laserscope can be safely used on all skin colors, and even after sun exposure. Similar lasers include the Candela GentleYAG.

For one full day after laser hair removal, you should refrain from exercise, the steam room, or anything that causes your skin to flush. You should also avoid the sun—especially sun bathing—for a few days. The treated hairs may fall out within a few days, but it can take up to three or four weeks.

Depending on the part of the country you live in, charges for laser hair removal should range from $150 to $500 per facial area, per treatment.

LASER HAIR REMOVAL FOR BAD IMPLANTS OR TO COMPLETE BALDING FOR A YOUNGER, SEXIER LOOK

A final note: we've had the unfortunate experience of meeting with patients who were the victims of inexpertly done hair transplants. Their hairlines looked totally unnatural, with hairs of various diameters growing in every which direction and practically screaming: *botched hair transplant!*

Until laser hair removal, there was little these unfortunate souls could do, other than cover up with a hair-piece. Today, it takes only one or two treatments to completely and permanently remove the badly transplanted hair, leaving the patient to start over or try another option.

As for partially bald men who prefer the sexier all-skin look, laser treatments can complete your baldness, eliminating the need for tedious and sometime painful daily shaving of the head.

The bottom line is that today's hair removal technologies can quickly and safely remove unwanted hair with minimal discomfort. Today, more than ever, going hairless is an easy and permanent option.

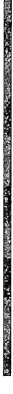

PART THREE

beauty
from head
to toe

chapter sixteen

beautiful teeth

O kay, you've had your wrinkles erased with Botox, your skin is smooth, thanks to CoolTouch and microdermabrasion, and you work out at the gym to keep your muscles toned and taut. But what about your teeth? The smile is the focal point of the face. While rejuvenating your skin, nose, and eyes will improve your appearance, these procedures may only serve to emphasize an imperfect or aging smile.

Teeth age too. Take a good look in the mirror. Have you noticed that your teeth have also grown older? An older smile is actually the reverse of a young smile. It shows less of the upper teeth and more of the lower teeth, because both lips lose muscle tone and begin to sag, covering more of the upper teeth and less of the lower. Other signs of aging teeth:

- **Front teeth are all the same length**. As we age, we tend to wear away the tooth enamel along the biting edges. Eventually, all the front teeth become the same length.
- **Dark teeth.** Eating abrasive foods, brushing your teeth, and natural wear and tear cause a reduction in the thickness of enamel, allowing more of the secondary layer of the tooth structure, the dentin, to show through. Dentin is normally yellow, with overtones of brown and gray. The thinness of the enamel allows these colors to show through more.
- **Discolored**, stained, or dingy teeth. Years of drinking tea, coffee, and cola, as well as smoking and certain medications, can lead to an older-looking, less than dazzling smile.
- **Chipped and cracked teeth.** Years of wear and tear often result in teeth that are chipped, cracked, and worn looking.

The good news is that you don't have to live with unattractive, aging teeth. Just as science has devised new methods to rejuvenate your face and skin, dental science has developed new dental materials and procedures. Your teeth can easily be lightened, brightened, and reshaped. Correct use of these new dental techniques can even improve the fullness and symmetry of your lips.

making your teeth look younger

Since we aren't dentists and don't perform dental procedures ourselves, we regularly suggest that our clients visit their dentists to complete their makeovers. We have asked Marc Lowenberg, D.D.S., a cosmetic dentist in New York City, to give us the latest word on what is available and how these products and procedures work.

BLEACHING

This is a relatively new and popular way to achieve a bright, white smile. You can have it done professionally or do it at home, although the professional results are noticeably better, because the solution used is stronger.

In-office bleaching. Also known as power bleaching, this can be done with either an argon laser or a plasma arc light. First, your dentist will apply a gel of 30 to 35 percent hydrogen peroxide directly to the tooth or teeth to be bleached. You will be asked to wear protective goggles, and the dentist will then activate the laser or arc light, which accelerates the action of the gel. Depending on the degree of discoloration of your teeth, you will require from one to three treatments. Each treatment takes approximately one and a half hours.

The majority of people don't experience any discomfort during power bleaching, except for the jaw fatigue involved in keeping the mouth open so long. However, a small percentage of patients with very sensitive teeth report discomfort or pain from the bleach itself. In these cases, the dentist will simply stop the procedure. The patient may then elect to try at-home bleaching.

The cost range for in-office bleaching, depending on the part of the country where you have it done, is approximately $500 to $1500. Generally, power bleaching needs to be repeated about every two years.

At-home bleaching. This requires use of a special plastic mold, customized by your dentist, that fits over your teeth and that you fill with a solution of carbamide peroxide. Depending on the strength of the solution you use, you'll need to wear the mold from two to four hours or overnight. You should see brighter, whiter teeth within two or three weeks. As with power bleaching, you'll need to repeat the procedure within two or three years.

Over-the-counter bleaching kits. These kits can lighten your teeth to some extent, but as the molds are not custom-made, the results are less predictable. The Crest White Strips, currently advertised on television, also work,

---

Dr. Marc Lowenberg's Six Key Ingredients for a Sexy Smile

A sexy smile begins with healthy-looking teeth. Sometimes what we consider sexy changes with fashion, or depends on the taste of the viewer. Still, some sexy traits are universal, and these are the defining characteristics I have listed here:

- **Dazzling white teeth** (Christie Brinkley)
- **A wide, full smile showing all the teeth** (Julia Roberts)
- **The upper two front teeth longer than the others** (Claudia Schiffer)
- **A slight imperfection in the position of the teeth** (Nikki Taylor)
- **Teeth that look healthy** (Heather Locklear)
- **Teeth that support a pouty lip** (Kim Basinger)

though not so well as professional bleaching.

Note that none of the methods for bleaching, including in-office power bleaching, work on all teeth. Because of individual chemical makeup, some teeth are simply not susceptible to lightening.

BONDING

Bonding is a modern procedure often used to repair chipped or cracked teeth, or to close a space between two teeth. It can also be used cosmetically to cover the surface of stained, discolored, or crooked teeth.

To bond your teeth, your dentist first etches the enamel layer of the chosen tooth or teeth with a mildly acidic solution, then molds a composite resin or plastic paste onto the enamel. The material is shaped with hand instruments, then the resin is hardened with a high-intensity light. The bonded material is then shaped and polished using the drill.

Bonding is painless and usually doesn't require anesthesia, unless part of your tooth needs to be ground down for a more radical reshaping. It is relatively inexpensive, and even better, the results are immediate. What you see is what you get—a bright new smile! Bonding generally costs $200 to $600 per tooth.

The only downside to bonding is that it is not as long-lasting as some other methods of cosmetic tooth repair. The bonding material can chip or stain fairly easily, and it is opaque, rather than translucent, like tooth enamel or porcelain, so it does not achieve quite the same degree of aesthetic beauty.

VENEERS

Porcelain laminate veneers are the Rolls Royce of cosmetic dentistry. With virtually no drawbacks, this technique provides a long-term solution for discolored, misshapen, old-looking teeth. Veneers correct a multitude of imperfections: they can change the color or shape of your teeth, actually making crooked teeth look straight; they can close gaps or spaces; they can lengthen worn-down teeth; and they can make the dental arch wider, giving greater support to your lips and cheeks, thus creating a fuller smile.

Veneering is an extension of the bonding process, and requires two office visits. In the first visit, the dentist will inject your gums with a numbing agent and use a drill to shape and slightly reduce the tooth structure. He then will take an impression to fabricate the veneers. At the second visit, usually a week or two later, he will etch the entire surface of the tooth and the inside of the laminate, then bond them together using a composite resin under a high-intensity light.

If you can afford them, veneers offer the best cosmetic result. The beauty and strength of porcelain is unmatched, and its translucence gives it a truly life-like appearance. Also, porcelain doesn't stain the way composite resin does, and it has a much more beautiful luster. Furthermore, porcelain lasts—an average veneer will still look good in ten to twenty years.

The cost range for veneers, depending on where you have them done, is approximately $500 to $2,200 per tooth.

Caring for Aging Teeth

Just as you pay more attention to your skin care regimen as you grow older, you should also concentrate more on how you care for your teeth. Growing older used to mean the inevitability of dentures, but no more. Today we understand enough about oral health that most of us can usually keep our teeth for a long and healthy lifetime.

According to the American Dental Association (ADA), it's increasingly important to keep your teeth and gums clean as you grow older, because plaque—the sticky bacteria that cause tooth decay and gum disease—builds up more quickly on the teeth of older adults.

The ADA offers the following guidelines for keeping your teeth--and keeping them healthy.

- Brush twice a day, using a soft-bristled brush and fluoride toothpaste. Always use products that carry the ADA Seal of Acceptance, which means that they meet the ADA's strict standards for safety and effectiveness.
- Clean between your teeth once a day, using floss or an interdental cleaner.
- Follow your dentist's recommendations for regular visits. For most people, that will be once or twice a year, but depending on your oral health, your dentist may want to see you as often as every three months.
- Eat a healthful, balanced diet, including foods rich in calcium and antioxidants.

COSMETIC CONTOURING

Cosmetic contouring, or reshaping, is an ideal treatment for very small cracks or chips, and can also be used to reshape your smile into one that is more pleasing. For example, if one front tooth is a little longer than the others, contouring can even them out.

While men's teeth tend to be angular and strong, often squared off, women's teeth are usually more attractive when the corners are rounded off. Since the natural process of aging flattens out the edges of the front teeth and tends to square off the angles, cosmetic contouring for women usually involves softening and rounding the teeth. Pointed canines, which sometimes have a vampire look, can also be rounded and softened.

To do contouring, your dentist uses a drill, sandpaper discs, and polishing wheels to gently reshape the targeted tooth or teeth. There is minimal loss of tooth structure involved, and anesthesia is not necessary. Once the treatment is finished, no further replacements or touchups are necessary.

The costs and time needed for contouring are minimal. The range for doing the entire mouth is approximately $150 to $500.

PORCELAIN JACKETS OR CROWNS (CAPS)

Crowns or jackets, commonly called caps, are a more complex and long-term solution for more complex problems, including major chips, very discoloured and misshapen teeth, and very worn and old-looking teeth. It's not uncommon, or example, for people in the public eye to have all their front teeth capped to hide imperfections and present a dazzling smile to the world.

The process for having caps made is similar to that for veneers, except that instead of slightly reducing the tooth's structure, the dentist will grind it down to a peg shape to fit inside the cap. At that first visit, an impression will be made and then a temporary cap will be fitted over the tooth.

A week to ten days later, you will return to the dentist's office to have the temporary cap removed and the permanent one put on with a bonding resin. The dentist or his assistant will hold the permanent cap tightly against your tooth while the bonding material hardens.

Permanent porcelain caps look beautiful—often far more so than your natural teeth. Judy, a fifty-eight-year-old patient, recently decided to cap her four top front teeth, which were not only very stained and worn, but of different lengths and widths. When fitting the permanent caps, the two center teeth

How to Find a Good Cosmetic Dentist

Although your family dentist may be a wonderful person and a terrific dentist, he or she doesn't necessarily have the skill and artistic eye necessary to create beautiful new teeth. We recommend searching for a dentist with specialized training and background in cosmetic procedures and the experience and aesthetic sense to create the ideal smile you seek.

When looking for someone, it's best to start close to home: ask your friends and colleagues for references, as well as your family doctor and dentist. Other places to search include the Yellow Pages and the Internet (see links to cosmetic dentistry in Appendix B). When you have some likely candidates, check them out in person.

A reputable cosmetic dentist should offer a free consultation. As you would when choosing a surgeon (see page 102), don't hesitate to ask about the dentist's background, the procedure, and what you can expect. Important points to check:

- Are the dentist's offices clean and comfortable?
- Do staff members (and the dentist) treat you courteously?
- What is the dentist's background? How long has she been in practice? Is the major part of her practice in cosmetic dentistry? A qualified dentist will be glad to share this information with you.
- How often has the dentist has performed the procedure you want? If the answer is evasive, the dentist may not have the experience you want for this procedure.
- Can you see before and after pictures of the procedure you are considering? If a dentist doesn't keep before-and-after photos, he probably doesn't perform cosmetic dentistry often.
- Can you contact patients who have had the same procedure done? A fully qualified, reputable cosmetic dentist should have no problem in sharing this information.
- Does the dentist offer you more than one option for the same results? Does he fully explain the differences?
- Does the dentist try to pressure you into receiving more treatment than you want? Never agree to extra treatments without a second opinion.
- Be sure also to ask about full costs, insurance coverage, and financing. Most cosmetic dental offices can help with insurance, if applicable, and offer some sort of financing.

were narrowed very slightly, while the outside teeth were slightly widened, to achieve a more aesthetic balance.

"I can't believe it!" Judy exclaimed after seeing the permanent caps. "My teeth have never looked this good before in my entire life!" She reported later that she finds herself smiling far more often than in the past, and that several people, including a new boyfriend, have commented on her beautiful smile.

The biggest drawback to caps is that the procedure requires removing a large portion of the tooth. It is the most invasive of all cosmetic procedures. In nearly all cases, veneers can be done instead, preserving more of the tooth structure. One exception is that any tooth that has been capped previously can only be re-capped.

Another drawback to permanent porcelain caps is their cost, which, depending on the part of the country where you live, can range from at least $750 per cap to more than $2,000.

chapter seventeen

beautiful
hands
and feet

If the skin on your face and neck have gotten wrinkled and spotted, it's a sure bet that the signs of aging are apparent on your hands and feet as well. Most of the treatments we've described for your face, neck, and chest can also be applied to your hands and feet, as well as some extra rejuvenation tricks we'll detail in this chapter.

hands-on solutions

By the time you reach middle age, your hands have been through a lot. They've dealt with sun, wind, rain, cold, heat, and harsh chemicals. They've worked hard and they usually show it, with thin, wrinkled skin, prominent blue veins, sometimes swollen knuckles, and a scattering of freckles and age spots.

Even worse, your hands have that bony look. The nice, youthful padding on the backs of the hands grows thinner as we age, revealing bare-seeming tendons and bones.

No matter how young your face looks, if your hands look old it's a giveaway of your calendar age. What to do? Luckily, there are a number of rejuvenating treatments that can quickly restore your hands to the suppleness and beauty of youth. Not only can your aging skin be made smooth, new treatments can also diminish bulging veins and that bony appearance.

TOPICAL SOLUTIONS

In earlier chapters we recommended tretinoin (Renova), glycolic acid, Kinerase, and a variety of over-the counter products including retinol to rejuvenate the skin. Just as these preparations can help to fade age spots on your face and neck, they work beautifully on your hands to help restore a more youthful appearance. The skin on hands that have been treated will appear thicker and less wrinkled, and any spots will disappear or be less noticeable.

Please note that whatever treatments you choose, it is *extremely* important to wear 30 SPF or higher sunscreen on your hands whenever you go out into the sun. Some of the treatments (tretinoin, glycolic acid) can increase your sensitivity to sunlight; in any case, past exposure sunlight is a big part of the reason that your hands look so bad now. Many products formulated for hands contain sunscreens, but they may not be strong enough if you are planning to spend a great deal of time outdoors.

The following are among the many topical products you can use to improve the appearance of your aging hands. For more on these preparations, including the suggested strength of active ingredients, see chapters 3 and 10.

Furfuryladenine (Kinerase). Just as Kinerase can improve the skin on your face, chest, and neck, it works wonders on the backs of your hands. Use once or twice daily, and be sure to apply sunscreen afterward.

Glycolic acid preparations. There are a number of prescription-strength and over-the-counter AHA and glycolic acid products formulated specifically for hands. Regular use should lead to a marked reduction in brown spots and minor wrinkling. Among the brands you may want to try are MD Forte; Foot Facial (available through our web site); Neutrogena; ROC; and Avon.

Retinol treatments. A number of over-the-counter retinol creams and lotions are formulated specially for the hands. As with retinol products for the face, these are not as strong as tretinoin, but regular use of these products should make a visible difference in the appearance of age spots and fine lines. Companies that make retinol creams or lotions for hands include Avon, RoC, and Neutrogena.

Renova. Renova, the prescription tretinoin cream that works wonders on your face and neck, can also greatly improve the appearance of your hands. You'll need to apply it to the backs of your hands at night before bed, since use with other products (such as sunscreens) can inactivate it. Also, because Renova causes photosensitivity, it's even more important to use an SPF 30 or higher sunscreen during the day. Some patients find that Renova causes irritation to the thin, delicate skin of the backs of the hands; try using it only two or three times a week, alternating with glycolic acid or another rejuvenating treatment.

INJECTABLE IMPLANTS

As we have said, the main reason aging hands look bony is because the natural fat padding beneath the skin on the backs of the hands has disappeared, leaving the veins and tendons prominent. Although it's not yet a widely performed procedure, small amounts of injectable implants, injected into the flat areas between the tendons on the backs of the hands and just above the wrists, can restore a youthful contour to the hands. Among the injectables used are Artecoll, Restylane, and autologous fat (for more information on these and other implants, see chapter 5). At the present time, hand implants generally last a few months before new injections are necessary.

LASER TREATMENTS

Lasers and IPL provide the most modern and fastest way to rejuvenate the hands. The Aura laser or Ruby, Alexandrite, and YAG-erbium lasers can quickly get rid of age spots and freckles, while CoolTouch II laser treatments can help to improve the skin texture as well as reduce wrinkling and the appearance of bulging veins and prominent tendons.

Vein therapy. The veins on our hands become particularly visible with age because the veins lose elasticity, allowing more blood to pool in them. At the same time, the fat padding beneath the skin has decreased and the skin has become thinner and more translucent, making the veins even more obvious. You may also have a hereditary tendency toward large, distended veins.

As with unsightly veins on the legs and other parts of the body, both sclerotherapy (see chapter 8) and laser treatments can reduce or eliminate their prominence. These newer sclerotherapy techniques, using milder injection solutions, are very effective for veins on the hands (as well as the legs). These new techniques work faster, pose fewer risks of side effects, and involve fewer needle sticks. To find a practitioner to perform sclerotherapy on your hands, look for a cosmetic plastic surgeon or other doctor who specializes in rejuvenation treatments.

PEELS AND MICRODERMABRASION

Superficial peels and microdermabrasion can also improve the appearance of the aging skin on your hands. Be sure to discuss all possible treatments with your physician, and bear in mind that, as with rejuvenating the face, a combination of treatments often produces the best results.

If your hands have not yet started to show age, we strongly advise you to begin now to protect them with sunscreen. Wear gloves when doing heavy or dirty work, and consider beginning a regimen with copper or vitamin C cream to maintain your natural collagen and smooth skin.

how to have gorgeous (yes, gorgeous) feet

Like your hands, your feet take a beating throughout life. Not only can they become unsightly, they can also be painful, due to a number of changes caused by lifestyle choices and simple aging. But unlike most of the changes due to aging that we have discussed in this book, not all changes to your feet are harmless. Some, in fact, can be the sign of a more serious problem, such as diabetes, vascular disease, arthritis, or a degenerative joint disease.

An ounce of prevention can definitely pay off in healthier and better-looking feet. Only buy shoes that fit, no matter how fashionable or sexy they are. Keep your toenails clean and trimmed, straight across rather than curved on the sides. Keep your shoes and socks clean and dry. By your forties and beyond, it's extremely important to consult a podiatrist about any problems you are having

Fingernail and Toenail Beauty Tips

Surprisingly, many people have more beautiful nails as they get older—thicker can be better. However, proper nail grooming is even more important as we age, to minimize any imperfections. Nicely groomed nails and cuticles, along with neutral colors, look good at any age.

For an expert opinion, Deborah Hardwick, founder and co-owner of BuffSpa at Bergdorf Goodman, gave this advice: Be sure to keep your nails properly trimmed. Healthy nails that extend just past the tip of the finger are the most youthful and the most fashionable—always. Long talons usually look dated.

Let the sides of your nails grow till they reach the end of your finger or toe. Then shape the top rather than filing down the sides. This makes the nail beds look longer and more beautiful, and keeps nails stronger. If you constantly break or snag your nails, shaping your nails this way will make a big difference.

Cut your cuticles only when needed, and train yourself to quit picking or biting them.

As for color, don't let yourself get into a rut. If you have certain colors that you always wear, consider *evolving* your favorites, not a radical change. Your nail technician will have ideas and be honest with you about what is flattering. So ask!

Some people do fine with home care for nails, but most people find that regular manicures and pedicures can educate them about nail care and greatly improve the look of their hands and feet.

However, if you use manicure and pedicure salons, the most important feature to check is hygiene. If the place doesn't look clean (floors, tables, benches, etc.), it isn't clean. Implements should undergo a medical-grade sterilization. Orange sticks and nail files should be for your use only, then thrown away.

Bringing your own implements is dangerous unless you are sterilizing them. Most germs are airborne, and proper sterilization is your only defense against a serious infection.

with your feet. The time and money you invest will be well repaid with healthier feet and perhaps a healthier overall body.

As for the cosmetic problems we see in aging feet, the most obvious are ugly toenails, bunions, calluses and corns, and distended veins and spider veins. These difficulties can lead in turn to a further cosmetic problem, the inability to wear flattering shoes. Luckily, all of these difficulties can be corrected easily and, in most cases, quickly.

UGLY TOENAILS

As you get older, your toenails (and to a lesser extent fingernails) naturally thicken. This thickening (technically, onychauxis) is caused by repeated trauma (too-tight shoes, too much walking on hard surfaces), circulation changes, and even poor nutrition. The problem may very well be complicated by a fungal nail growth (onychomycosis), which is quite common in damaged nails.

FUNGUS

We've seen some women patients who simply cover the problem up with nail polish, but without treatment this simply allows the nail damage and fungus to get worse. Besides, thickened, distorted toenails don't look much better under a coat of polish than they do bare. It's certainly not a bad idea to disguise the problem with (usually dark) polish when your feet need to be seen, but treatment will work better if your nails are bare.

Fungus is most likely to grow in toenails that have previously been injured. You can help protect them by avoiding places where fungus like to hang out, such as improperly sterilized foot baths or implements at nail care salons, or bare gymnasium floors (wear flip-flops). When having a pedicure or a manicure, make sure that the salon passes our "look-test:" if it doesn't look clean, walk out; if, while waiting, you don't see the operators opening sterile instruments and changing the water in the foot-bath, walk out.

If you already have a fungus (the nail will darken or become very yellowed; it may also appear thin and flaking or crumbly), topical antifungal drugs, such as Penlac and Restore, can help. Although oral drugs also exist, we prescribe them as a last resort because of the possibility of rare side effects. Most important is to regularly visit and follow the advice of your podiatrist. Eventually, the fungus will clear and you will be proud once again to show off your bare feet.

YELLOW TOENAILS

If you don't have a fungus, but your toenails are nevertheless thick and yellow, the best thing you can do (besides making sure that all your shoes fit) is to visit your podiatrist and have her file them down; she may even use a grindstone on any particularly distorted nails. She can also recommend a whitening agent to help restore your nails to their natural color.

If you have badly discolored toenails (or fingernails), be aware that podiatrists can perform bleaching treatments. Also, at-home regular soaks in hydrogen peroxide keep nails less yellow and are a good hygiene practice. Simply pour the peroxide into a bowl straight from the bottle (or use a cotton ball to saturate nails) and soak for two to five minutes. After peroxide quits bubbling, it turns to water.

CORNS AND CALLUSES

Corns and calluses are both caused by friction, usually from shoes. Corns appear on the tops of your toes (or occasionally between the toes), while calluses appear on the ends of your toes, the balls of your feet, and sometimes your heels. Corns are smaller than calluses; they are generally the size of a pea or smaller, and have a hard, conical center that grows into the skin. Because they usually appear directly over bone, corns are often quite painful, while calluses are generally painless, but unsightly. Both are basically hard, horny layers of skin that your body creates in an attempt to cushion your bones from pressure or rubbing.

The best way to avoid calluses and corns is to choose shoes that fit well. For shoes you will be walking, playing sports, or hiking in, make sure that there is a thick, cushioned sole and a high, roomy toe box (so the tops of your toes don't rub the shoe when you walk). For recurring corns and calluses, your podiatrist may need to prescribe an orthotic, a specially fitted shoe insert that redistributes your weight more evenly, preventing any one area from receiving too much pressure. At our web site (see Appendix B) you can buy a fashionable OrthoChic insert that will provide many of the benefits of a custom-made orthotic, but costs much less and is much more stylish. To get rid of calluses:

- Use a pumice stone or emery board after a bath or shower for small calluses that aren't causing pain. Gently rub the built-up area, taking care not to damage the adjacent skin.

  NOTE: Never use sharp instruments. Never cut into calluses, which could cause an infection.

- Microdermabrasion, which is primarily used on the face (see chapter 3), provides a gentle and effective way to get rid of large areas of callused skin, as on the heel or ball of the foot. Preceded by a mild chemical peel, this is one of the best ways to eliminate large areas of thickened and yellowed skin, revealing new, beautiful, and supple skin beneath. The procedure is painless and relaxing. Five to ten treatments are usually recommended, at one per week.

- Depilatories. An over-the-counter depilatory (such as Nair), when applied to calluses (not corns!) for five to eight minutes, will make it easier to rub the excess skin away.
- Bear in mind that glycolic acid lotions and other products for hand and body care can also improve the appearance of the skin on your feet. (See Appendix B for recommended Foot Facial Products).
- After soaking in lukewarm water, use Dr. Levine's Fabulous Foot Facial Kit (see Appendix B to order) or create your own: use a mild exfoliant (such as an 18 percent glycolic acid preparation), a foot masque with salicylic acid, a pumice stone, and complex mineral moisturizer to help collagen formation.
- Always see a podiatrist if the callus becomes reddened or acutely painful, which can indicate infection.

To get rid of corns:

- Although they usually can't get rid of corns, corn pads and rings, as well as moleskin cut to fit, can help cushion the affected area and reduce pain, as well as prevent the corn from getting worse. They do not, however, relieve the underlying cause of the corn, which can be due to a muscle imbalance and hereditary factors.

     Over-the-counter corn-removal products contain caustic substances, such as salicylic acid, that gradually soften the thickened skin. This material must be applied carefully because it will irritate the adjacent normal skin. You'll know when you apply it incorrectly because the adjacent skin will burn and hurt. As you age, the skin becomes thinner and the risk of irritation and pain greater.
- Sometimes soaking your corn, then filing away the excess tissue with an emery board or pumice stone, can provide relief.

   NOTE: Never use sharp instruments. Never cut into corns, which could cause an infection.

- See your podiatrist for recurring or painful corns. She will usually be able to remove them quickly and easily. In some cases you may need surgery to remove the underlying cause, such as a hammertoe. Your doctor can also prescribe orthotics, if needed, and will tell you if you need a different style or bigger size of shoes (probably you do).
- Always see a podiatrist if the corn becomes reddened or acutely painful, which can indicate infection.

SPIDER VEINS AND SMALL VARICOSE VEINS ON THE ANKLES AND FEET

No matter how gorgeous your new strappy sandals, they will not look good if your ankles and feet resemble a roadmap of prominent veins and/or spider veins. These ugly purple and reddish lines are usually the result of heredity, hormones, pregnancy, or simply too much standing. As with problem veins elsewhere on the body, modern procedures offer quick and relatively painless permanent solutions.

- Laser treatments. One to three nearly pain-free sessions with the Lyra or Aura laser will often zap those unsightly veins for good. (For more information on treatment of veins by laser, see chapter 6).
- Injection sclerotherapy. As with varicose veins or unwanted veins anywhere else on the body, injection sclerotherapy can erase those ugly veins with minimal discomfort and expense. (For more information, see page 91). Follow-up treatments are often necessary, involving another injection sclerotherapy procedure or a combination treatment with a laser.

BUNIONS

Bunions are not only unsightly, they can be acutely painful. These twisted, gnarled knobs, usually found on the side or top of the big toe joint, are the result of improper foot biomechanics, usually from years of ill-fitting shoes combined with a hereditary tendency. Often, the only shoes that offer relief are sandals, but nothing looks uglier than a bunion bulging through delicate straps.

A bunion is actually an arthritic degeneration within the joint of the toe. It affects the toe itself, causing it to twist inward and press against the next toe, sometimes moving under or over it (a condition called hammer toe). Adding

If you are diabetic

All foot problems are more serious for diabetics because of compromised circulation to the foot. If you are diabetic, don't treat your own feet. Especially *do not* use over-the-counter corn and callus products. You may have decreased sensation of pain in your feet and may not notice irritation from the caustic ingredients in these products, resulting in damage and infection. All foot treatment should be performed under sterile conditions; see your doctor for the treatment of corns, calluses, bunions, and other foot problems.

insult to injury, bunions and hammer toes can cause rubbing of your feet against your shoes, resulting in corns and calluses.

Unfortunately, home and over-the-counter remedies provide only temporary relief. If the pain is not too severe, the following measures may help:

- Have your podiatrist prescribe custom orthotics, which help stabilize the foot, provide some relief, and slow the progression of the bunion.
- Always wear properly fitting shoes. Try a larger size than you now wear; especially look for a larger toe box.
- Wear sandals.
- Soak your feet in warm (not hot!) water with Epsom salts for fifteen minutes (follow the directions on the package).
- Alternatively, soak your feet in vinegar water (one capful of vinegar to one gallon of water).
- Ice applied to an acutely painful area may help; take care if you are diabetic not to over-chill the area.

Although many bunions can be managed indefinitely with the above measures, in some cases the deformity or pain becomes disabling, and the only permanent solution is surgery. This should be provided only by a podiatrist or orthopedist who specializes in foot surgery.

A number of new procedures can reduce the bunion without hospitalization, using minimal incisions and local anesthesia. The bunion will be gone, the bump vanished, and the toe straight. You will walk out of the same-day surgical center in a special shoe. Full recovery takes no more than six to eight weeks.

You think high heels are sexy and show off your legs and feet to their best advantage. Unfortunately, it has become too painful to wear heels except for very short periods of time. Must you resign yourself to a choice between burning agony on the balls of your feet or living forever in clunky, unflattering flats?

painful soles

Until fairly recently, the answer to that question was "yes." The basic cause of the pain was loss of collagen and fat padding in the ball of your foot. Adding extra padding to the shoes sometimes helped, but the problem inevitably grew worse. Today, however, thanks to CoolTouch and similar lasers, your doctor can zap the bottoms of your feet and induce new collagen to grow, replacing the lost padding.

Because the skin on the sole of your foot is thicker than other skin, and is also often callused, the callused skin will first be removed with multiple means. The area will then be treated with ultrasound, which will provide a pleasant warmth. Immediately afterward, the CoolTouch laser will be used to activate the collagen-producing cells just under the skin. An injectable implant, such as collagen, might then be injected under the skin.

There's no downtime, and the new collagen stimulated by the laser begins to fill in within six to eight weeks. A number of patients who have had this procedure are once again gadding around town in their Manolo Blahniks. (For more on CoolTouch, see chapter 6.)

MORTON NEUROMA

Morton neuroma is an acutely painful inflammation of the nerve sheath between two toes, usually the third and fourth (between the second and third is the next most common). While anyone can develop this condition, it is most common in women, with the incidence peaking at about age sixty. Men can get it at any age. Morton neuroma is caused by irritation of the nerve, possibly from ill-fitting shoes. Runners and dancers have a particular predisposition to Morton neuroma because of the extra and unusual stress they place on their feet, though anyone can get it.

The CoolTouch laser can provide some relief of the pain and burning on the bottom of the feet that commonly accompany this condition. Treatment includes laser, ultrasound therapy, and sometimes the injection of filler material, similar to that used for cosmetic purposes.

Anita, in her early fifties, is a well-known ballerina and teacher of ballet who suffered an injury to her right foot ten years ago. "You know dancers," she said ruefully. "We just won't stop after an injury." Instead of taking time off to rest, Anita continued to give performances and to teach.

She ignored the pain in the balls of her feet, even when they started feeling numb. After examination, it was clear that Anita had developed Morton neuromas on both feet. Though this isn't an uncommon problem, it had been made worse by the years of dancing and wearing high heels, which had eroded the natural padding on the balls of her feet.

We agreed together to try CoolTouch II treatments, to stimulate her own collagen, supplemented with a small amount of injected collagen until her own new collagen could begin to form, and therapeutic ultrasound.

After six weeks of treatment, Anita was pain-free and remains so with the help of CoolTouch II touchups (every six months or so) and moleskin padding that she sticks to the balls of her feet when she dances or wears high heels. "I'm so happy to still be able to wear heels," she said. "After all, as an artist, I'm an ambassador of culture. I have many roles to play and want to look my best."

SUN-DAMAGED FEET

Although your feet are not usually as damaged by sun exposure as your hands and face, ugly freckles and brown spots, as well as wrinkles, can show up here too. All of the procedures mentioned earlier for hands work equally well for the delicate skin on your feet.

HAIRY FEET

Although hairy feet aren't usually a problem for women, they can be quite unsightly on men. Hairy toes, hairy tops—many find this excessive hirsuitism very unsightly. If you'd like to eliminate or at least reduce the hairs on your feet so you'll look better in sandals, laser treatments provide a quick and relatively painless solution. The laser treatments we described in chapter 15 are just as effective on the feet; check with your podiatrist for a referral to a doctor experienced in laser treatments.

Suzanne Levine's Tips for Healthy Feet

- **Prevention** is the number one way to protect your feet. Avoid walking or dancing on hard or uneven surfaces. Never wear thin soles on bumpy ground. And never wear ill-fitting shoes—even for a special occasion.
- **Get plenty of exercise.** This will strengthen the feet themselves as well as improve your overall circulation. The most beneficial exercise is walking, at least thirty minutes a day.
- **Don't go barefoot** if you have any sort of neurological problem or diabetes; you could easily pick up a cut that you don't feel. Infection is also a danger.
- **Wear supportive, well-fitting shoes** for your walk. Jogging shoes are particularly good.
- **Watch out for obstructions** as you walk.
- **Only walk where the lighting is good.** Remember that your eyes are getting older, too!

---

chapter eighteen

eating for health and beauty

It may not be true that you are what you eat, but as you grow older, your appearance can mirror your diet. When you are very young, you can get away with skipping meals, gorging on junk food, and ignoring supplementation. Not so as you grow older. Your metabolism is slower, especially after forty, and every calorie you consume should count in terms of nutrition.

We're not going to lecture you here on filling up with veggies rather than cookies, or get into the controversy of low-carb versus high-carb diets. But we do want to stress the ways in which your diet affects the way you look as you age.

how your weight affects your appearance

It's true that we all tend to get heavier as we get older; that's not necessarily a bad thing, as long as we don't gain too much weight. The sylph-like looks of a teenage model are actually inappropriate for a woman of fifty because her body needs some extra fat, both to replace some of the hormones that are lost at menopause (fat tissue produces small amounts of both female and male hormones) and because the added weight can help keep her bones strong. Besides, too-thin often translates to gaunt, which is very aging and reveals every line and wrinkle.

The converse, too much fat, is aging too, partly because we tend to associate excess weight with a matronly appearance in women and with middle-aged flab in men. Besides, when you're obviously overweight there is a tendency to low self-esteem and neglecting the rest of your appearance. Instead of doing what they can to look youthful and vibrant, many overweight people, even those who are only carrying a few extra pounds, tend to give up and opt for shapeless clothes and utilitarian makeup and hairdos.

Unfortunately, most of us don't realize that we are putting on pounds every year as our metabolisms slow until we wake up one morning thirty pounds overweight and with a paunch, spare tire, and double chin. Not only is the fat itself aging, but when you lose the weight your skin can sag and fold, making you look even worse. The folds are not only unsightly, they can become infected.

CoolTouch treatments can help some with saggy skin, but usually the only solution for excessive skin is some form of plastic surgery.

Obviously, the best solution is to avoid gaining weight in the first place, or to lose it as soon as it becomes noticeable. The following guidelines from our colleague, Eva To, a registered dietician, can help.

DIET AND WEIGHT LOSS TIPS

- Eat balanced meals: starches (rice, bread, pasta, potatoes, corn), protein (lean meat, fish, poultry, low-fat dairy), and fiber (cooked or raw vegetables, salad, fresh fruit). Minimize fats.
- Eat every three hours. Do not skip or delay meals. Take a protein bar with you at all times. If meals are delayed, eat the snack first.
- Beware of hidden fats: fried foods and snack foods, salad dressings, regular cheese products, oils, butter/margarine, mayonnaise, gravies, pesto sauce,

cream soups, and sauces. Beware of hidden sugars: fruit juices (fresh or frozen), sodas, iced tea, lemonade, fruit punch, "smoothies," non-fat desserts, and regular desserts.

• Eat fresh fruits and vegetables daily.
• Avoid alcohol on an empty stomach.
• Try not to snack on high-calorie foods at night.
• Drink eight (yes, eight!) glasses water daily unless you have a kidney problem. That's 64 to 80 fluid ounces a day. Carry a water bottle with you. Water helps our kidneys to function properly, gets rid of toxic waste in our system, keeps our complexion clear, and helps with weight maintenance by making us feel full. It also keeps skin supple and naturally moisturized.
• Try to walk or at least move after each meal for five to ten minutes.

vitamins and your skin

In chapter 10, we discussed the use of topical vitamins to retard and reverse signs of aging on the skin. Taking the right supplements orally can also help your skin's appearance, but beware of hype. Too many Americans want to believe that they can find eternal youth in a jar or bottle. The American Academy of Dermatology offers guidelines in choosing vitamins to protect against and reverse aging.

Bear in mind that vitamins—the right vitamins—are only part of the story. Even more important is sun protection. Work with a dermatologist to devise the right program for your own lifestyle and skin type. Also, be sure to tell your doctor about other medications and supplements you are taking, to avoid harmful interactions.

Among the supplements that can improve your appearance are the following:

• **Selenium** The mineral selenium is a proven cancer-fighter, including sun-induced skin cancers. It also helps prevent oxidation-caused changes to the skin, which result in loss of elasticity. Dietary sources of selenium include whole grain cereals, seafood, garlic, and eggs. A typical oral dose of selenium would be 50 to 200 micrograms.
• **Vitamin E** As we discussed in an earlier chapter, vitamin E is the oil-based antioxidant that protects cells throughout the body. In addition to offering topical sun protection, there is evidence that oral supplementation with

vitamin E helps protect the skin against sun damage. Dietary sources include vegetable oils, especially sunflower oil; grains such as wheat germ, brown rice, and oats; nuts; dairy products; and meats. A typical supplement of vitamin E would be 400 IU (international units), taken with food.

- **Vitamin C.** This vitamin is the most abundant antioxidant found naturally in the skin. As a potent antioxidant, vitamin C protects the skin from sun and other environmental damage, including smoke and pollution. It helps prevent skin cancers and slows aging changes. In chapter 10, we recommended topical vitamin C for skin rejuvenation. Vitamin C supplements in your diet can further protect your skin, as well as improve your immunity and the health of other body systems. Good dietary sources of vitamin C include most vegetables and all citrus fruits. A typical recommended level of vitamin C supplementation would be 500 to 1000 milligrams a day.

Before you start on any vitamin regimen, check with your doctor, especially if you regularly take prescription or over-the-counter medications, because vitamins can sometimes interfere with the effectiveness of certain drugs.

chapter nineteen

exercise: the magic bullet

W e hope we've persuaded you that using the treatments and products we recommend in this book can help you maintain the best possible look as you grow older. However, even if you've had Botox and CoolTouch for your wrinkles, laminates for your teeth, and an updated hairdo appropriate for your age and facial structure, there's no way you can look your best without taking care of your body as well.

We know you've heard it all before—that keeping your body active will keep it looking its best. In this chapter, we hope to convince you that exercise truly is "the magic bullet" for appearance as well as health. The truth is that beginning an exercise program at any age truly does provide virtual "age reversal," even after years of sedentary living. If you're already a confirmed exerciser, good for you! On the next few pages you can check our recommendations to see if you're doing the right kind of exercise to maintain a healthy skin, bones, and figure.

the unwelcome stranger in the mirror

As we mentioned in the chapter on diet, our metabolism slows down as we age. In our thirties and forties, we may not notice it so much because we are so busy and active with family life and career, but from about the mid-forties on, body muscle begins to be replaced with fat, which is a double whammy. Not only does fat take up more space on the body than lean tissue, causing those formerly well-fitting trousers to bulge in unwanted places, but fat takes fewer calories to maintain than muscle, so the more fat you have, the fatter you get.

The fact is that an exercised, well-toned body looks better in all types of clothes—and without them as well. No, you cannot regain the body of a teenager, but we have clients in their fifties who declare that they are in better physical shape than they were when they were teens.

Besides delivering a trim body, exercising will also improve the appearance of your complexion and your hair by improving the circulation and delivering more oxygen to all tissues. Regular exercise also relaxes you, leading to a calmer and more rested (and therefore youthful) overall demeanor.

The advantages of exercise are not just a question of appearance, of course. We're sure that you have heard the evidence linking inactivity with various diseases, including heart disease, diabetes, and some forms of cancer.

We can usually tell long-term exercisers when they appear in our office because they seem to have more energy and a more positive outlook on life. But even beginning for the first time in later years can have tremendously beneficial consequences.

Take fifty-five-year-old Donna, an executive secretary, who had always been attractive, but became dissatisfied with her appearance and her life. She came to us for Botox treatments to erase the worry lines around her eyes. Though thrilled with the results, Donna confessed that she had not only noticed aging changes in her face, but her body had begun to resemble "a stranger that barely fit in the mirror." Renewing the beauty of her face was easy for us, but we explained that rejuvenating her body was up to Donna.

Although she was sure that she would never be able to stick with a program, Donna joined a health club on our advice.

"I realize now that I have to work at what used to come without effort," she told us several months after our first meeting. "I now have two Jims in my life," she added, showing off her newly svelte figure. "One is my long-term beau, James. The other is G-Y-M, my new three-times-a-week companion. I walk every day and then work out for an hour and a half at the gym. It's work. It's hard. It's tiring. But it's necessary, and I will never give it up."

Before you begin an exercise program (or update your current one), you need to be sure that it includes three basic components. Each of the components is important and each will rejuvenate your body in a different way.

for your heart: aerobics

Aerobic exercises are the ones most of us think of when we imagine sweating and grunting: those exercises that raise your heart rate, cause you to break out in a sweat, and cause you to breathe more quickly. Aerobic exercises are essential to the health of your heart and lungs. They also improve your appearance by improving your circulation, delivering more oxygen to all your body's tissues, and they increase your metabolism, thus helping you to lose or keep off weight.

The most popular aerobic exercises are jogging, aerobic dance, step aerobics, Stairmaster, cycling, and swimming. One of the best of all aerobic exercises is walking, which can be done any time and anywhere. The most important things to remember about aerobic exercises are that they must be done at a rapid enough pace to raise your heart rate (test: you should be able to sing to yourself or carry on a conversation, but your breathing should be faster than when you're just resting), and they must be performed for a sufficient amount of time to work out your cardiovascular system, a minimum of twenty minutes at a time, three to five times a week.

for your body: strength training

Strength training exercises are those that specifically build muscle mass. They are performed by working your muscles while using weights, but the weight can be simulated (as with rubber band exercises) or provided by your own body, as with yoga and some kinds of calisthenics.

It used to be believed that strength training was necessary only for people who had to do a lot of heavy lifting in their work or for bodybuilders, but it's now known that everyone, of all ages, can benefit from strength training. By building muscle, you'll increase your overall metabolism and protect all the joints in your body. More important is that strength training helps to protect your bones from osteoporosis (as do weight-bearing aerobic exercises like walking). Strength training also helps make everyday life easier—no more problems opening stuck pickle jars! Best of all, strength training will greatly improve your appearance, reducing flab and building muscle, improving your posture, and increasing your stamina for sports or simply daily living.

You're never too old for strength training, by the way. Studies have been done on seniors as old as their nineties, and it's been found that a simple weight-training program can significantly increase their strength and muscle mass, improving quality of life.

The most popular strength training exercises are weight training, using free weights (dumbbells and barbells) or workout machines such as Nautilus and Cybex; isometric exercises, in which one set of muscles is pitted against another; and calisthenic-type exercises, such as the Canadian Air Force exercise program, Pilates (exercise with an emphasis on stretching and strengthening muscles), or vigorous forms of yoga (Power Yoga, Ashtanga Yoga).

Note: before beginning a weight training regimen, be sure to work with a personal trainer, take a class, or follow a tape. When working with weights, correct form is very important, and must be observed to prevent injuries.

for your lifestyle: flexibility and balance

Flexibility—being able to move your joints freely and without pain—and balance are components of fitness that impact the quality of your life. The more flexible you are (within limits), the less likely you are to injure yourself when performing other exercise or engaging in sports. Also, the easier everyday life will be. Balance helps you move with grace and also prevents falls, which can be a serious problem the older you get, resulting in broken bones and a restricted lifestyle.

The best exercises for improving flexibility and balance include such Eastern systems as yoga and T'ai Chi, and Pilates.

You may believe that you are too old to benefit from exercise, but we want to assure you that starting now, or improving your current exercise program, can only have positive benefits in your life. In our opinion, you can't afford *not* to exercise.

If you've been exercising for a while, but feel you are no longer receiving the benefits, you may want to consider interval training, which involves interspersing very intense periods of exercise with less vigorous periods. For example, if your regular aerobic exercise is walking, you might want to mix in short bursts of power walking or even jogging.

Our colleague Eva To, a registered dietician and fitness counselor, tells about Betty, a fiftyish client who was trying to lose weight for her son's wedding, but she had plateaued, finding it impossible to lose more than five pounds.

First, Eva To had Betty split her exercise into morning and evening sessions of shorter duration. Then she taught Betty how to do interval training by playing with the speed and incline buttons on her treadmill, and added weight training three times a week. After six months, not only had Betty reached her goal weight, she announced that she had picked out a dress for the wedding, and it was a size 6.

starting an exercise program

If you are new to exercise, or are just beginning again after a long period of being sedentary, the following guidelines will help make it easier:

- Check with your doctor before you embark on any exercise program.
- Don't exercise on an empty stomach, which can actually lower your metabolic rate. Eat a snack before exercise, or wait 30 minutes after a meal to do intense aerobic exercise.
- Avoid boredom by cross-training: try different forms of aerobic exercise, and add interval training by varying the speed of walking or the intensity of exercise.
- Consult with a physical trainer or use exercise tapes or a guide book for proper strength training techniques.
- Find a workout buddy, especially if you have trouble making yourself exercise. Whatever you're doing—walking, aerobics, weight training—is easier when you have someone to share it with.
- Remember that you're never to old to improve your health and appearance with exercise. Studies show that men and women in their nineties have improved their balance and increased leg strength after starting an exercise program.

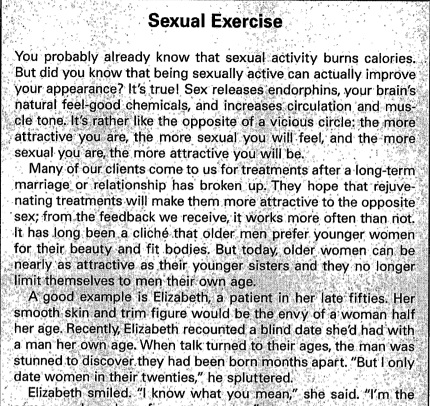

Sexual Exercise

You probably already know that sexual activity burns calories. But did you know that being sexually active can actually improve your appearance? It's true! Sex releases endorphins, your brain's natural feel-good chemicals, and increases circulation and muscle tone. It's rather like the opposite of a vicious circle: the more attractive you are, the more sexual you will feel, and the more sexual you are, the more attractive you will be.

Many of our clients come to us for treatments after a long-term marriage or relationship has broken up. They hope that rejuvenating treatments will make them more attractive to the opposite sex; from the feedback we receive, it works more often than not. It has long been a cliché that older men prefer younger women for their beauty and fit bodies. But today, older women can be nearly as attractive as their younger sisters and they no longer limit themselves to men their own age.

A good example is Elizabeth, a patient in her late fifties. Her smooth skin and trim figure would be the envy of a woman half her age. Recently, Elizabeth recounted a blind date she'd had with a man her own age. When talk turned to their ages, the man was stunned to discover they had been born months apart. "But I only date women in their twenties," he spluttered.

Elizabeth smiled. "I know what you mean," she said. "I'm the same way. I much prefer younger men."

chapter twenty

attitude

As we said back in chapter 1, old isn't old anymore. Or at least, it doesn't have to be. Throughout this book we've showed you the latest products, treatments, and lifestyle changes you can use to turn back the hands of your personal clock. You may choose to try one, or several, or none of them. But we hope that we have helped to show you that aging is more than a matter of years. If you want to remain youthful, you can—as long as you retain a youthful attitude.

Societal norms are changing. It's no longer considered strange for a grandmother (or grandfather) to ride a motorcycle, or for a woman of seventy to play three sets of tennis before lunch. The old saying that you're only as old as you feel has become literally true in the twenty-first century.

No longer do we need to give up and give in to growing old. No longer do we need to try too hard to look younger, making ourselves ridiculous in the process. Instead, through our lifestyle choices and care for our skin, hair, and body, we can remain truly young for many years past middle age.

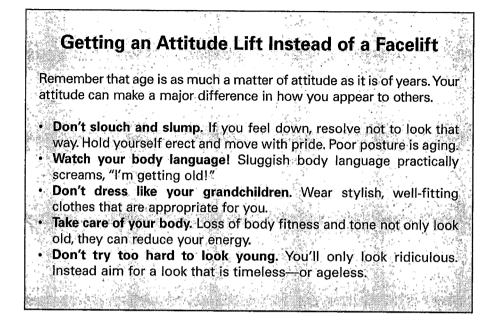

Getting an Attitude Lift Instead of a Facelift

Remember that age is as much a matter of attitude as it is of years. Your attitude can make a major difference in how you appear to others.

- **Don't slouch and slump.** If you feel down, resolve not to look that way. Hold yourself erect and move with pride. Poor posture is aging.
- **Watch your body language!** Sluggish body language practically screams, "I'm getting old!"
- **Don't dress like your grandchildren.** Wear stylish, well-fitting clothes that are appropriate for you.
- **Take care of your body.** Loss of body fitness and tone not only look old, they can reduce your energy.
- **Don't try too hard to look young.** You'll only look ridiculous. Instead aim for a look that is timeless—or ageless.

glossary

Actinic keratosis (plural: keratoses)—A flat, dry, rough, or scaly spot with a reddish appearance. These blemishes should always be examined by a doctor, as they may be precancerous.

Alpha-hydroxy acids—Natural fruit or milk acids used to smooth skin and reduce blemishes and minor wrinkling.

Antioxidant—A substance that prevents the damaging effects of oxygen in body tissues.

Autologous fat—Fat that is taken, by liposuction, from one part of the body to be used in another part.

Beta-hydroxy acids—Natural plant acids, such as salicylic acid, used alone or with alpha-hydroxy acids to smooth skin and reduce blemishes.

Botox—A substance made from botulinum toxin used to relax muscles. Botox is used for various medical purposes as well as to improve appearance.

Collagen—The structural material that gives skin its plumpness and resilience.

CoolTouch laser—A medical laser that restores natural collagen and improves the texture and appearance of the skin.

Dermis—The middle layer of skin where collagen and elastin originate.

Elastin—The structural material that gives skin its elastic properties.

Epidermis—The outer, protective layer of skin, comprised of dead skin cells.

Fibroblasts—Specialized cells in the skin's dermis that produce collagen and elastin.

Free radicals—Unstable molecules produced by reactions with oxygen or pollutants that in excessive amounts can cause tissue damage in the body.

Glycolic acid—A widely-used form of alpha-hydroxy acid derived from sugar cane.

Humectant—A cosmetic ingredient that attracts moisture to the skin.

Hyaluronic acid—A natural component of the skin that is used as a biodegradable injectable filler.

Hyperhidrosis—Excessive sweating.

Injectable implants—Materials (usually liquid or gel) that are injected into the skin to fill in scars and wrinkles or otherwise plump out sunken areas. Commonly used injectables include Artecoll, Reviderm, Restylane, Rofilan, Perlane, New Fill, collagen, silicone, Dermologen, and Gore-Tex.

Intense Pulsed Light (IPL)—A medical device that produces intense broad-spectrum light to stimulate the formation of collagen, which will improve and even out skin color and texture.

Keloid—An enlarged scar that projects above the skin surface.

Laser—A machine that produces a beam of concentrated light used for industrial and medical purposes. Medical lasers can improve or erase discolorations and unwanted growths, as well as stimulate production of skin collagen and elastin. Most lasers are used for one specific purpose, such as removing unwanted hair. Commonly used lasers include the YAG-erbium (CoolTouch), the I-Nd:YAG (Aura), and HeNe (Nlite).

glossary

Liposuction—A medical procedure in which unwanted fat is removed from beneath the skin.

Lipstick lines—Small vertical lines that appear above the mouth.

Marionette lines—Furrows that extend from the corners of the mouth to the chin.

Melanin—The dark pigment that gives skin and hair their color.

Melanocyte—A specialized cell that produces melanin.

Microdermabrasion—A nonsurgical procedure that removes dead cells from the surface of the skin, revealing a fresher and clearer complexion.

Myobloc—A substance made from botulinum toxin used to relax muscles. Like Botox, Myobloc is used for various medical purposes as well as to improve appearance.

Nasolabial folds—Deep furrows that extend from the corners of the nose to the corners of the mouth.

Orthotics—Custom-made shoe inserts that are designed to correct a mis-alignment or other foot problem.

Pattern baldness—A type of hereditary baldness in which hair falls out in a distinct pattern, such as on the crown, leaving a horseshoe-shaped fringe of hair.

Peel—A skin rejuvenation treatment that removes part of the outer skin. Peels can be chemical (such as alpha-hydroxy) or mechanical (such as microdermabrasion). Light peels remove only the outer layers of the epidermis; deep peels remove the epidermis and parts of the dermis.

Platysma muscle—The wide, flat neck muscle that with age separates into prominent strands, leading to "turkey neck."

Retinol—A precursor to tretinoin, an acne treatment derived from vitamin A.

Rosacea—A skin condition of unknown cause in which large portions of the face become abnormally red.

Sclerotherapy—A nonsurgical treatment to get rid of unwanted bulging or varicose veins.

Seborrheic keratosis (plural, keratoses)—A generally harmless, warty, raised, brown or yellow spot caused by age and sun exposure.

Senile lentigo (plural: lentigenes)—Benign flat brown spots caused by age and sun exposure; also known as "liver spots" and "age spots."

SPF (sun protection factor)—A rating that indicates the degree of sun protection offered by sunscreens, sunblocks, and sun-protective clothing.

Telangiectasia—Red or purple blotches caused by broken or enlarged blood vessels beneath the skin.

Tretinoin—A derivative of vitamin A that can prevent and even heal sun damage to the skin. Brand names include Retin-A and Renova.

UVA, UVB—Ultraviolet A and B are the two types of sunlight that cause sun damage to the skin, leading to premature aging and even skin cancer.

YAG-erbium—A type of cosmetic laser.

appendix a
for further reading

The following books offer more information on several of the issues we discuss in this book.

Cooper, Kenneth. *The Aerobics Program for Total Well-Being: Exercise, Diet, Emotional Balance*. Bantam Doubleday Dell, New York, 1985.

Lautin, Everett M., M.D., Levine, Suzanne M., D.P.M., and Lance, Kathryn. *The Botox Book: What You Need to Know About America's Most Popular Cosmetic Treatment*. M. Evans and Company, Inc., New York, 2002.

Levine, Suzanne M., D.P.M. *My Feet Are Killing Me!* Fawcett Crest, New York, 1987.

Nelson, Miriam E., Ph.D., with Wernick, Sarah, Ph.D. *Strong Women Stay Slim*. Bantam Books, New York, 1998.

Nelson, Miriam E., Ph.D., with Wernick, Sarah, PhD. *Strong Women Stay Young*. Bantam Books, New York, 1997

Voltage, High. *Energy Up!* Perigee, New York, 1999.

appendix b

web

sites

general information and shopping

Many of the products we recommend in this book, such as Kinerase, are distributed through doctors only. However, unless they are prescription products they can usually be found on the Internet (on doctors' and other medical sites), where they may be somewhat less costly than those sold in a doctor's office. Be aware, however, that shipping costs can add greatly to the overall purchase price. By all means use a browser to compare prices and get the latest information on new rejuvenating products. Some of the sites with particularly good information include:

Institute Beauté. This site, maintained by the authors of this book, offers information and a wide range of selected products to enhance and preserve your appearance (and your feet).

http://www.institutebeaute.com/

Part of the Altruis Biomedical Network, this site offers information on all aspects of health care, including extensive information on cosmetics.

http://www.cosmetic-information.com

The American Academy of Dermatology maintains this web site, which offers tons of information on all aspects of skin care.

http://www.aad.org/

The American Board of Medical Specialties (ABMS) can help you determine if your surgeon is certified. To connect to their Online Certification Verification Database:

http://www.abms.org

The American Dental Association maintains an excellent site with information on all aspects of dental care.

http://www.ada.org/

The American Society of Aesthetic and Plastic surgeons offers extensive consumer advice on all aspects of cosmetic enhancement, including up-to-date information on all procedures as well as a search engine for locating a plastic surgeon in your area.

http://www.surgery.org/default.htm

American Sun Protection Industry is a nonprofit organization representing manufacturers of sun-protective products. Lots of good info on this site.

http://www.americansun.org

web sites

iEnhance is a web-based community of patients, health care providers, and suppliers, offers a wide range of information on all aspects of aesthetic treatments, including a locator service for aesthetic physicians by area.

http://www.ienhance.com

IVillage is a comprehensive web site devoted to topics of interest to women. It contains a great deal of useful information on cosmetic products and procedures, as well as other health and medical information.

http://www.ivillage.com

A huge, comprehensive web site about male pattern baldness. Lots of info on all treatments, as well as support, chats, and sales of various products.

http://www.regrowth.com

The Skin Cancer Foundation, a clearinghouse for information about skin cancer causes, cures, and prevention, offers a wealth of info on skin changes to look out for, how to pick a sunscreen, and much more.

http://www.skincancer.org

Information on collagen treatments.

http://www.aesthesticsurg.com

Information on products for soft tissue augmentation.

http://www.artecoll-usa.com

Information on skin repair and rejuvenation.

http://www.canderm.com

This web site by the aerobics pioneer Kenneth H. Cooper offers books on nutrition, exercise, and stress reduction, and sells vitamin formulations for various lifestyles.

http://www.cooperwellness.com

Paula Begoun, the "Cosmetics Cop," offers a number of useful cosmetics-related articles on this web site, which also sells beauty products and Begoun's beauty-related books.

http://www.cosmeticscop.com

Skin products and services.

http://www.dermalive.com/en

This informative website is maintained by fitness guru High Voltage.

http://www.energyup.com

Information on products for restoring hair growth.

http://www. finasteride.com

Information on a variety of hair treatments, including Nioxin hair products.

http://www.hairsite.com

Information on breast implants and collagen injections

http://www.lnamed.com

Explains the benefits of collagen treatment

http://www.isolagen.com

Offers very low prices on Kinerase and a number of other skin products. For some products, this site offers the price to beat.

http://www.kinerasedr.com/policies

Tissue transplantation

http://www.lifecell.com

Vivienne Mackinder, internationally known hair stylist and makeup expert, maintains this site, which offers information on makeup and hairdos and sells various beauty education products.

http://www.mackinder.com

MD Forte's products.

http://www.mdforte.com

Information on laser eye surgery.

http://www.nidek.com

Q-Med Esthetics products available in Canada.

http://www.restylane.com

This site, home of Rofil Medical International, offers information on its products Reviderm, Rofil, and Artecoll.

http://www.rofil.com/

Studio Five specializes in beauty products and makeup for men.

http://www.studio5ive.com/

"Cosmetic Yellow Pages" offers a wide variety of beauty-oriented products and services.

http://www.topdocs.com

One of the most informative sites on the Web, maintained by a woman who has had multiple cosmetic procedures, this site serves as a kind of clearinghouse for all varieties of cosmetic procedures from creams to surgery. Marianne, the site's proprietor, has pulled together a variety of medical and lay sources, as well as her own experience with the products and procedures she has tried. The site also includes chats and bulletin boards. Highly recommended.

http://www.yestheyrefake.net/index

The following sites are among dozens on the Internet that offer tips on avoiding sun exposure as well as a complete line of sun-protective clothes for the whole family:

http://www.sunprotectiveclothing.com/

http://www.solareclipse.com/

http://www.thepinktree.com/UV_protection_faq.htm

Aboutcosmeticdentistry offers information on all aspects of cosmetic dentistry, as well as a dentist locator service.

http://www.aboutcosmeticdentistry.com/

The web site of Dr. Dominic A. Brandy offers extensive information on surgical and other solutions to baldness.

http://www.brandymd.com/

The Connecticut Children's Medical Center has a good fact page on cerebral palsy and Botox, including contact information for patients' families and doctors.

http://www.ccmckids.org/departments/Orthopaedics/orthoed18.htm

This excellent site is operated by Audrey Kunin, M.D., a dermatologist who provides excellent information on cosmetic products and procedures and also sells products.

http://www.dermadoctor.com/

The Dystonia Foundation maintains this web site, which offers a great deal of information on the various forms of dystonia and its treatments. Click on

http://www.dystonia-foundation.org/nsda/treatment/reimburse.asp

for a direct link to a page explaining The Botox Advantage, a program offered by Botox maker Allergan to help patients get insurance reimbursement for medical Botox treatments.

http://www.dystonia-foundation.org/

The American Electrology Association offers information on electrolysis and an online search engine for board-certified electrologists.

http://www.electrology.com/

Canadian doctors Marvin Schwarz and Brian Freund have been conducting ongoing studies on the use of Botox to treat TMJ disorders. For more information, check out their very informative web site.

http://www.max-facial.com/index.htm

The World of Hair is an excellent, extensive online reference by Dr. John Gray, provided by the P & G Hair Care Research Center.

http://www.pg.com/science/haircare/hair_twh_12.htm

Dr. James J. Romano, a San Francisco plastic surgeon, maintains this site, which explains the huge number of plastic surgery (and non-invasive) options for rejuvenation of the entire body, including hands. Dr. Romano includes a special section on rejuvenation for men.

http://www.jromano.com

smoking cessation sites

Freedom From Smoking Online is the American Lung Association's free quit-smoking program, which offers tips, support, and links through a series of "modules."

http://www.lungusa.org/ffs/index.html

Christine H. Rowley, the host of this About site, offers a wide variety of arti-cles on smoking and quitting, including tips of the day and discussion forums and chat.

http://quitsmoking.about.com/

This site offers links to the latest drugs and counseling techniques for treating tobacco use and dependence.

http://www.surgeongeneral.gov/tobacco/

appendix c

professional

articles

Abulghani, A. A., Shirin, S., Morales-Tapie, E., Sherr, A., Solodkina, G., Robertson, M., Gottlieb, A.B. "Studies of the effects of topical vitamin C, a copper binding cream, and melatonin cream as compared with tretinoin on the ultrastructure of normal skin." *Journal of Investigative Dermatology*. 110 (4); 1998.

Agerup, Bengt. "An explorative study on the histology following one year of implantation of Zyplast and Restylane in normal skin." Abstract. *Q-Med Sweden.*

Anderson, R. Rox. "Lasers and their clinical applications." In *Current Challenges in Dermatology*, Upjohn, November, 1991.

Biddle, Jeff E., and Hamermesh, Daniel S. "Beauty, productivity and discrimination: lawyers' looks and lucre." *J Labor Economics;* 1998 Jan (16:1): 172–201.

Binder, William J., Blitzer, Andrew, and Brin, Mitchell F. "Treatment of hyperfunctional lines of the face with Botulinum toxin." *A Dermatol Surg.* 1998; 24 (11): 1198–1205.

Bousquet, Marie-Therese and Agerup, Bengt. "Restylane lip implantation: European Experience." *Operative Techniques in Oculoplastic, Orbital, and Reconstructive Surgery.* Vol. 2, No. 4. December, 1999, 172–176.

Brandt, F. S. and Bellman, B. "Cosmetic use of botulinum A exotoxin for the aging neck." *Dermatol Surg.* 1998 Nov; 24 (11): 1232–1234.

Carmichael, Robin L, R.N., "Copper complexes in skin care products." In *Proceedings of the Fourth International Symposium on Cosmetic Efficacy.* May 10–12, 1999, New York.

Carruthers, Jean D.A. and Carruthers, Alaistair. "Botulinum toxin and laser resurfacing for lines around the eyes." In *Management of Facial Lines and Wrinkles*, Blitzer, A. et al., eds., Lippincott, 2000. chapter 20: 315–332.

Duranti, Fabrizio and Salti, Giovanni. "Different forms of hyaluronic acid gel in the treatment of facial wrinkles." Abstract. *12th International Congress on Aesthetic Medicine.* November 1999.

Goldberg, David J. "Non-ablative subsurface remodeling: clinical and histological evaluation of a 1320-nm Nd: YAG laser." *Journal of Cutaneous Laser Therapy.* 1999: 1: 153–157.

Hamermesh, Daniel S. and Biddle, Jeff E. "Beauty and the labor market." *Amer Econ Rev.* 1994 Dec. (84:5): 1174–1194.

Jackson, Edward M., Ph.D. "The importance of copper in tissue regulation and repair: a review." *Cosmetic Derm.* 10: 10 Oct. 1997: 35–36.

Nauman, M., Hofmann, U., Bergmann, I., Hamm, H., Toyka, K., and Reiners, K. "Focal hyperhidrosis: effective treatment with intracutaneous botulinum toxin." *Arch Dermatol.* 1998 Mar: 134: 301–304.

Newman, James. "Nonablative laser skin tightening." *Facial Plastic Surgery Clinics of North America. Minimally Invasive Surgery.* Vol. 9, number 3. August 2001.

Olenius, Michael. "The first clinical study using a new biodegradable implant for the treatment of lips, wrinkles, and folds." *Aesth Plast Surg.* 22: 97–101, 1998.

Pham, Randal Tanh Hoang Pham. "Nonablative laser resurfacing." *Facial Plastic Surgery Clinics of North America. Facial Rejuvenation: Nonsurgical Modalities.* Vol. 9, Number 2. May 2001.

Pons-Guiraud, A. "Non-animal stabilized hyaluronic acid (NASHA) as dermal filler for wrinkles and lips treatment." *EADV*, September 1999.

Spencer, James M. "Cosmetic uses of botulinum toxin type B." *Cosm Dermat.* 2002 Feb: 15 (2): 11–14.

West, T. B. and Alster, T. S. "Effect of botulinum toxin type A on movement-associated rhytides following CO2 resurfacing." *Dermatol Surg.* 1999 April (25): 259–261.

index

217

index

index

about the authors

Everett M. Lautin, M.D., F.A.C.R., a graduate of Columbia College and Downstate College of Medicine, State University of New York (SUNY), former professor at the Albert Einstein College of Medicine, has been practicing medicine for more than thirty years. Dr. Lautin frequently lectures throughout the United States and abroad on non- and minimally invasive medical rejuvenation. He has been interviewed on this subject for articles in magazines and newspapers such as *Vogue, Glamour, New York Magazine,* the *Times* magazine (London), the *New York Times, Concorde, The Evening Standard* and *Marie Claire.* Dr. Lautin has given television interviews on WNBC, WABC, KOMO, Fox News, and Metro TV. He is the author of numerous articles in the medical literature and medical textbooks, and letters in the *New York Times* and *Discover.* This is his second trade book.

Suzanne M. Levine, D.P.M., a graduate of Columbia University and New York College of Podiatric Medicine, has been practicing podiatry for more than twenty years. Dr. Levine is the author of five books, including *Your Feet Don't Have to Hurt, My Feet Are Killing Me, 50 Ways to Ease Foot Pain,* and *The Botox Book* (with Dr. Lautin). Dr. Levine is frequently interviewed for articles in such publications as *US Weekly, Elle, Glamour, Woman's Day, Vogue, W, Shape, Allure, Newsweek, Family Circle, Ladies Home Journal, New York Magazine, USA Today,* the *New York Post,* the *Wall Street Journal,* the *Times* (London), and the *New York Times.* She is also a familiar presence on television and has appeared on *Today, The View, Weekend, Today in New York, Fox and Friends, The Oprah Winfrey Show,* and *Live with Regis and Kathie Lee.*

Drs. Everett M. Lautin and Suzanne M. Levine are the physician-owners of Institute Beauté (http://www.institutebeaute.com), a medical center on New York's Park Avenue, which provides head-to-toe rejuvenating medical treatments, and Institute Beauté Inc., the teaching arm of their practice, which provides instruction and guidance for physicians involved with rejuvenation treatments.

.